SCOPE® MONOGRAPH ON

The Fundamentals of
OPHTHALMOSCOPY

DAN M. GORDON, M.D., F.A.C.S.
Clinical Professor of Ophthalmology
Cornell University Medical College

PUBLISHED BY THE UPJOHN COMPANY, KALAMAZOO, MICHIGAN

Editor/Baird A. Thomas

Table of Contents

PREFACE

It is the purpose of this monograph to teach the beginner some of the fundamentals of ophthalmoscopy. The material included is intended for use by medical students and physicians who will not be practicing ophthalmology. It incorporates some of the lectures which I have given to medical students in ophthalmology over the years. I have attempted to make this monograph clinically applicable and free of much of the theory which I myself have found difficult to understand as a student and later as a practitioner.

This book is not intended to teach diagnosis of ophthalmic intraocular diseases; it is far too small for that purpose. Many diseases of the retina and choroid are described in a rapid fashion, only in order that the reader will be able to apply their use to the illustrations and to fundi which he examines. The reader who wishes to go further into ophthalmoscopy is referred to many of the more comprehensive texts on the subject; some of which were utilized by the author in preparing this book. The fundus photographs are from my private collection and the eye department of the New York Hospital-Cornell University Medical Center. I am grateful to the publishers for permitting the use of so many colored illustrations; and like every author, I would have liked to have quadrupled the number of pages and illustrations.

Dan M. Gordon, M.D.

EDITOR'S NOTE:

It is with great regret that we report that Dr. Dan M. Gordon died unexpectedly September 17, 1970, while recovering from an operation.

It will indeed, be difficult for Dr. Gordon's many friends, as it is for us, to realize that his energetic and enthusiastic efforts for the betterment of the practice of ophthalmology are at an end. It is, we believe, characteristic of him that in spite of his illness he completed the final details for this book just a few days before his death so as not to delay its production.

Since we could not have the benefit of his help with the final proofs, we have done our best to see to it that this final effort of his shall do him honor.

Fig. 1
Hand ophthalmoscopes.

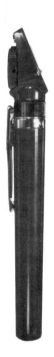
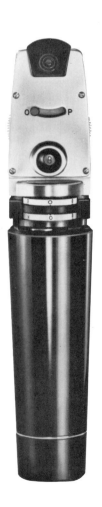
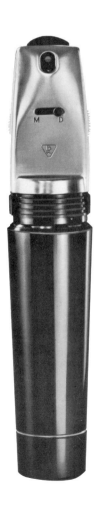
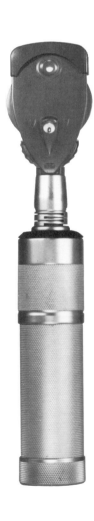

The Fundamentals of
OPHTHALMOSCOPY

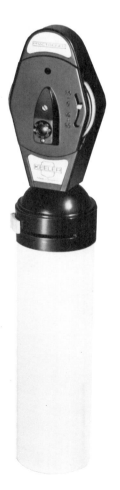

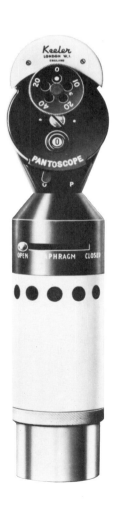

Introduction

The ophthalmoscope is one of the more important instruments in the physician's armamentarium. The results obtained from its use are dependent upon the quality of the instrument and the knowledge of the user. The best hand instrument is one which is electrified and connected to the wall via a transformer, which permits up to approximately 12 volts. This gives a most satisfactory light source, and is the best type of ophthalmoscope for office use. Most battery powered ophthalmoscopes give approximately 2 volts, and are satisfactory for the average purpose, while a transformer is a heavy object to carry around in a bag. It is necessary to employ fresh (or freshly charged) batteries with reasonably frequently changed bulbs, so that the brightest possible light is used. Inasmuch as the indirect method of ophthalmoscopy requires special skill and training, it is not described here.

Many hand ophthalmoscopes have varying devices for modifying the light projected; specifically two different sized round beams, a criss-cross grid, a vertical light stripe, and a round green light. It is wise to learn to use the ophthalmoscope with glasses if the latter are worn; employing a rubber guard on the instrument head for the purpose of preventing spectacle scratches. The head (usually a May type) with a disc, which contains a number of plus and minus (usually black and red) lenses ranging up to approximately 15 or 20 in power, may in the case of the electrified instruments contain accessory discs carrying additional lenses which permit employment of as much as plus

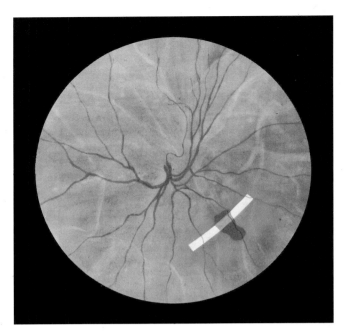

Fig. 2A
When the beam passes over a flat, non-elevated lesion it is not distorted.

Fig. 2B
When the beam passes over an elevated lesion (mass) the light is bent convexly towards the observer.

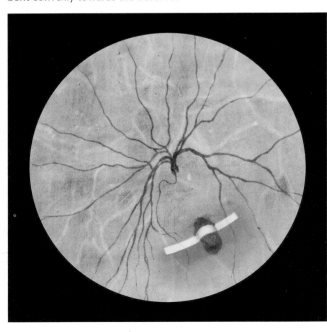

or minus 40 or more. If one is viewing the fundus of a patient who wears high-minus lenses, it may be wise to view his fundus through the patient's glasses, thus permitting the use of a low power lens in the ophthalmoscope. This procedure is rarely necessary in viewing high-plus fundi, which are usually found in aphakic individuals—aphakic without a lens; i.e. the cataractous lens has been removed surgically. Viewing the fundus through the patient's high-plus lenses creates too much distortion. Myopia (near sightedness) is neutralized ophthalmoscopically by the minus (usually red) lenses and hyperopia (far sightedness) by the (usually black) plus lenses in the ophthalmoscope.

The two differently sized round beams supplied by the ophthalmoscope are intended for small (undilated) and large (dilated) pupils respectively; in actual practice we become accustomed to using one or the other size routinely. The vertical slit (stripe) is for measuring or gauging convexity or concavity when viewing a retinal lesion. If the lesion is viewed with the slit beam, one of three impressions will be gained: (1) a flat lesion such as a hemorrhage, plaque or scar will not distort the slit, (2) an elevated lesion such as a tumor or fibrous mass will, when the slit is placed over both it and an apparently normal retina, cause a step-like distortion of the slit (fig. 2-B) with the convexity towards the observer, and (3) a depressed area such as a pit in the optic nerve, or the excavation in the nerve, or a true hole in the macula will, when the slit is placed over both the area surveyed and adjacent normal retina, cause the slit to be bowed away from the observer. The grid is to be employed to measure blood vessel size by placing the grid over the vessels and measuring the number of spaces required to measure a vessel calibre. It is rarely employed. The green beam is a red-free light beam for determining whether a black retinal "spot" is due to melanin or old hemorrhage. Unfortunately, the 2 volts supplied by the battery ophthalmoscope are insufficient for this purpose: but if the batteries are fresh some idea of the differential diagnosis may be possible. Employing red-free light with stronger voltage (i.e. 6-12 volts) old hemoglobin appears coal black and melanin much less black. Small aneurysms and hemorrhages (as in diabetics), which often are missed with ordinary illumination, will stand out sharply, black in color when the red-free light is employed. Obviously the blood filled vessels will also stand out as black stripes with the red-free light. Using red-free light makes it possible to trace the normal nerve fibers of the retina away from the optic nerve; conversely in optic atrophy since the nerve fibers are involved, the retina will appear somewhat marbleized. The red-free light is a most useful one, rarely appreciated because it is infrequently employed. Abnormal fundi should be viewed through both the traditional white or yellow light (which depends upon the bulb used) and the red-free light to gain experience with both available light sources. When possible the same fundus should be viewed through both a battery and a 12 volt instrument to illustrate the advantages of the latter.

Mydriasis (dilatation of the pupil) is necessary for complete examination of the fundus. Mydriasis is not to be confused with dilatation due to the use of a cycloplegic. A mydriatic such as 2.5-10% phenylephrine will dilate a pupil so that it will not narrow down markedly when the (up to twelve volt) ophthalmoscope light enters it; but will not permit sufficiently maintained dilation for fundus photography. Here it is necessary to paralyze the sphincter action of the pupil by using a cycloplegic (i.e. cyclopentolate), which is short acting but efficient. We often use a combination of both mydriatic and cycloplegic for more rapid dilation. When one completes his examination it is wise to instill one drop of 1 or 2% pilocarpine, followed by another drop 5-10 minutes later, to constrict the pupil. This is done to render the patient comfortable and ambulatory since the dilation affects his accomodation. Constriction militates against provoking angle closure glaucoma in individuals whose anterior chamber angles are shallow and hence readily closable. A general practitioner should not use a cycloplegic because he cannot evaluate chamber angle. In fact he probably should not dilate the pupil at all (legal involvement).

Ideally, the patient should remain in the examining room until the pupil has begun to constrict. In any event the patient should be instructed to phone or return if he suffers from unusual blurriness or pain. If this occurs, more pilocarpine should be employed every fifteen minutes until constriction begins, and two tablets of a carbonic anhydrase inhibitor (ethoxzolamide, acetazolamide or dichlorphenamide) should be taken. Instructions can be given by telephone, if necessary. In this same connection predetermination of whether it is, or is not, safe to dilate a specific patient is dependent, not upon his intraocular pressure but upon the depth of his anterior chamber angle. It is not always feasible to examine this by the use of a slit-lamp and contact lens; but it is possible to secure a good idea of its depth by gauging the depth of the anterior chamber. If this is of average depth, the patient is safe for dilation. Estimation is done in two ways: (1) by looking at a number of eyes until one acquires a fairly good idea of the average distance between the cornea and the iris, and (2) by casting a light such as that of the ophthalmoscope from which the head has been removed, onto one limbus and looking at the horizontally opposite limbus to see how far the base of the iris appears to be

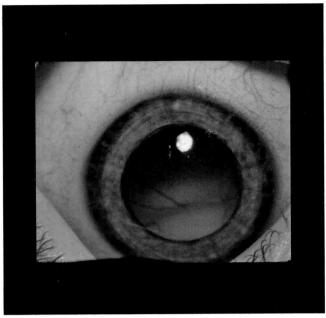

Fig. 3
This is the red reflex seen at a distance of several inches, employing high-plus lenses (approximately plus 15). One sees a thin veil containing dark retinal vessels—undoubtedly a retinal detachment.

Fig. 4A
A very cloudy media (vitreous) in a patient with severe uveitis. The observer sees only an orange area corresponding to the disc.

Fig. 4B
Red reflex in a patient with extensive acute choroiditis. The yellow part of the reflex of the field corresponds to the acute lesion.

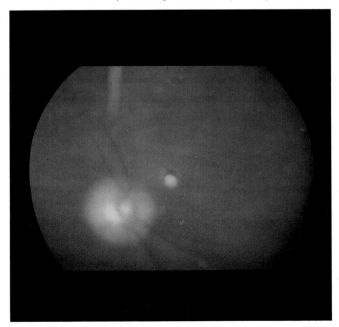

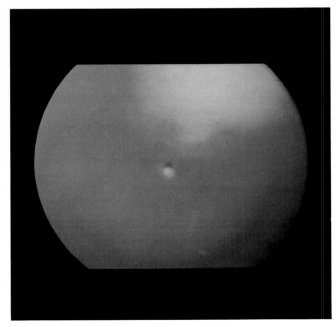

from the corneal limbus. If it appears to be virtually touching, consider it a shallow angle and dangerous to dilate. If one can see that it is not shallow, then it is not dangerous. If one must dilate and is uncertain, give the patient one tablet of a carbonic anhydrase inhibitor when dilation is initiated, and at least two successive (five to ten minutes apart) instillations of 2% pilocarpine after concluding the examination.

The ophthalmoscope should be considered as analagous to a monocular microscope, which means that one's accommodation must be relaxed during its use. The skilled ophthalmoscopist will relax his accommodation when viewing the retina; the novice knowing that the retina is only one inch away will focus about -7.00 diopters in accommodation in order to see retinal detail. Each number in the ophthalmoscope aperture represents that many diopters of plus or minus sphere; i.e. $12-12$ D. If the observer's accommodation is relaxed, the number in the aperture represents the total of his and the patient's spherical refractive error. If he has no refractive error or is wearing corrective lenses, the number represents the patient's spherical refractive error. If that number is plus 2 and the observer is unskilled, he is accommodating approximately -7 D; the patient's error is then plus 9 D; the skilled observer would use 9 D of ophthalmoscope power to visualize the patient's retina.

The direct (hand) ophthalmoscope gives a magnification of approximately fourteen times. Indirect ophthalmoscopy will not be discussed here. The latter gives less magnification than the direct method, but combined with pressure on the globe gives access to all of the retina, compared to the lesser area seen by direct ophthalmoscopy. There are various modifications of the hand ophthalmoscope which are more expensive and which expose a greater degree of the fundus to visualization, than does the conventional May type head with which we are all familiar. There are other nonportable ophthalmoscopes, such as the Gullstrand binocular ophthalmoscope, which will not be discussed, but existence of which should be known to the reader.

When one is about to perform ophthalmoscopy (often erroneously termed "funduscopy") he should turn the disc to plus 15 or 16, stand off about 12 inches, and pick up the golden red fundus reflex. With this lens he will obtain a magnified, fairly clear view of the cornea. If there is any opacity in the normally clear red reflex, one should attempt to determine it's nature. Any such opacity must be in or on the cornea, in the anterior chamber, lens or vitreous. Often one can observe in the red reflex the orange ball of the optic disc (the terms optic disc, nerve and papilla are synonymous) or the yellow-white area of a choroidal scar, or the dirty yellow area accompanied by myriads

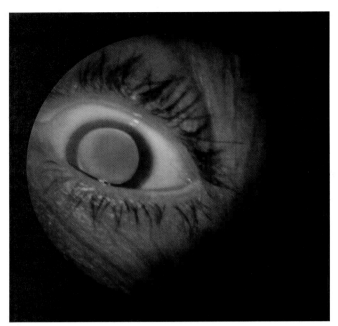

Lens changes as seen with the ophthalmoscope:
Fig. 5A Nuclear sclerosis—disc-shaped opacity

of tiny, black floaters signifying acute choroiditis. If the opacity is a corneal foreign body or scar it will be recognized by using the ophthalmoscope as a flashlight. Further, the corneal opacity will be nonmotile. Except for a lens dislocated into the anterior chamber, an anterior chamber opacity can be ruled out, as a lens practically always settles down out of sight into the lower part of the angle of the anterior chamber, unless it is so large that it will project up beyond the pupillary border. In the latter case, as well as in the event of a dislocated lens, the object will be seen grossly with the ophthalmoscope used as a flashlight. If the opacity is in the lens the appearance will depend upon whether the pupil is or is not dilated. Lens opacities (cataracts) tend to create one or a combination of three images: (1) a nuclear sclerosis or drying of the lens creates a round, translucent disc appearance, most obvious through a wide pupil, (2) cortical lens changes create pyramidal or streak-like black lines coming in from the periphery to invade the pupillary zone and (3) posterior subcapsular and the less commonly noted anterior subcapsular opacities create the appearance of a number of black dots forming a star-like or Christmas tree figure. Anterior and posterior polar cataracts, which are rare, cause a dense, small, round black opacity in the center of the pupillary zone. Vitreous hemorrhages replace the golden red reflex, so that their appearance depends upon

Fig. 5B
Cortical changes—pyramidal or linear shaped

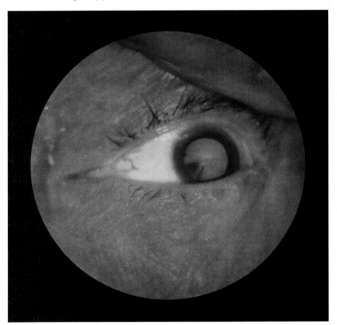

Fig. 5C
Posterior subcapsular cataract—a collection of dots forming an irregular, often Christmas-tree or stellate figure.

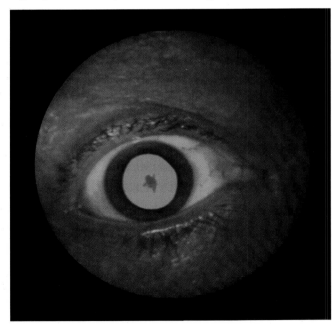

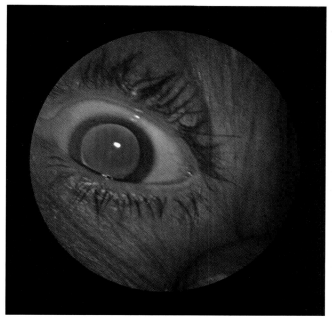

Fig. 6A
Nuclear sclerosis (nuclear cataract) in the red reflex, with pupil dilated. Note the central dark disc, corresponding to the large, sclerotic lens nucleus.

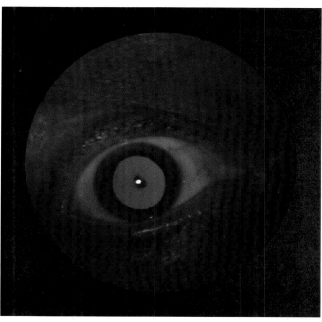

Fig. 6C
Posterior subcapsular changes in red reflex—appear as a black mass of dots.

Fig. 6B
Cortical spokes due to changes in the lens cortex. There are several pyramidal projections coming out from the pupillary border and pointing towards the center of the red reflex area.

Fig. 6D
Posterior polar cataract using the ophthalmoscope as a flashlight.

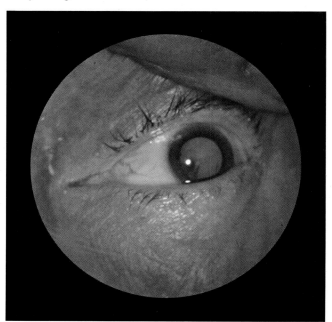

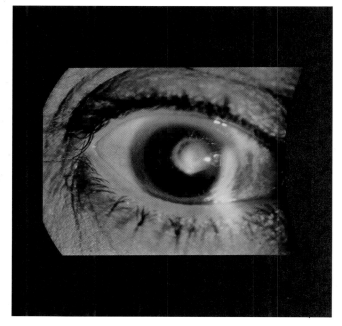

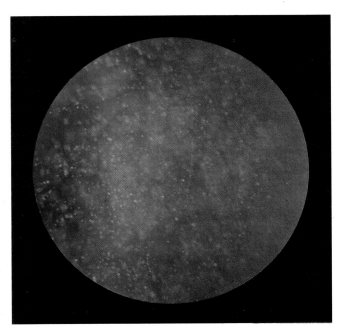

Fig. 7
Asteroid hyalitis. The vitreous is full of golden dots which move with motion of the globe and obscure observation of the retinal detail.

their size. Unless they are so huge as to completely replace the red reflex with a black one, vitreous hemorrhages will be noted as black motile opacities which move with motion of the eye. If they are so large that the fundus cannot be viewed, when the patient closes his eyes for a few minutes and then is examined before the eyes move actively, the hemorrhage may settle down sufficiently to permit a rapid examination of the fundus. If not, the patient should be put to bed with a backrest and both eyes bandaged overnight. The patient then is reexamined following dilating drops and the eyes rebandaged long enough for the drops to function.

After one has picked up the red reflex, and is still viewing it with a high-plus lens, he should ask the patient to rapidly look up, down, right, left and then straight ahead. If there are any floating foreign masses in the vitreous these will be seen. Large vitreous hemorrhages will appear as large floating masses, which tend to settle down. Small hemorrhages will be noted as chains of black cocci in the red reflex. Vitreous floaters (which may be pathologic, but usually are not) will be noted as small round black or linear spots floating about in the pupillary zone of the agitated eye. Transparent worm-like floaters are common in myopic individuals.

Vitreous hemorrhages frequently, and vitreous floaters rarely, are pathognomonic of underlying re-

Fig. 8A
A normal optic disc with a central physiologic excavation (lighter colored area) in which the truncated cone of emanating vessels is visible. The gracefully sinuous retinal vessels leave the disc at approximately one, five, seven and eleven o'clock.

Fig. 8B
A normal optic nerve head with a huge physiologic excavation, which might be mistaken for a glaucomatous excavation. Although wide and deep, it is surrounded by a normal rim of nerve tissue.

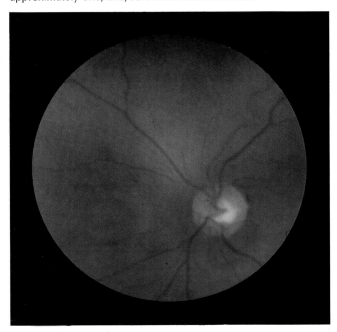

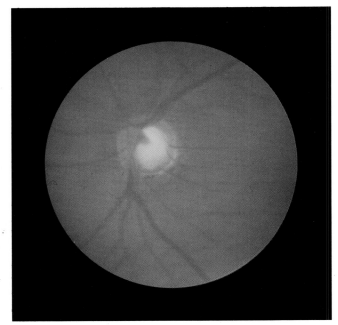

tinal detachments and indicate a search for the latter. If the observer notes gray or silvery areas elevated above the retinal level, he is viewing a detached retina until proved otherwise. The vitreous is a gel, which tends to become more fluid with increasing age and in myopia. It may even become detached so that one may see a large black ring floating in front of the red of the fundus itself—usually an annoying but not a serious situation, unless the vitreous is adherent to the retina, which it may then tear, producing retinal detachment. Occasionally one will see myriads of silvery or golden dots floating in the vitreous of one of the patient's eyes—denoting an asteroid hyalitis or synchysis scintillans. This is usually without great significance. It is due to various salts, such as cholesterol and represents a form of vitreous degeneration.

Having thoroughly examined the red reflex, the examiner will decrease the plus power and begin to approximate the patient's refractive error as he approaches the red reflex and begins to examine the interior of the eye. With the patient looking straight ahead at some distant target, with both of his eyes open, the optic nerve will be seen easily. This, in the normal eye is orange or reddish colored and may have a yellowish central excavation through which the central artery and vein enter and exit. There may be tiny dots as seen looking through a sieve in the bottom of the excavation, denoting the lamina cribrosa. Normally, the physiologic excavation will take up but a fraction of the surface of the disc, with the vessels bifurcating on its surface. Careful observation will indicate that there are a number of fine, threadlike blood vessels on the surface of the nerve, which do not cross from the disc to the retina, and which are the nutrient vessels of the optic nerve. If these are minimal or absent (especially if in contrast to the other normal disc) one is dealing with some stage of optic atrophy, in which case the disc will be yellowish or white in appearance. One should always compare the two fundi—as at least one is apt to be normal. If one excavation is larger than the other, that one should be viewed as glaucomatous until otherwise disproved. The physiologic excavation may be virtually nonexistent or may take up most of the disc area. In the latter event a normal rim of disc will be visible and the retinal vessels will cross the disc to exit at one, five, seven and eleven o'clock. In an advanced glaucomatous excavation, the glial framework is absent in the excavation, and cannot support any vessels which would be crossing the disc; hence these must go around the margin of the disc to exit temporally. As they exit from the disc as following the inner lining of a cup, one can see them bend sharply over the edge, in contrast to the flat appearance of norm-

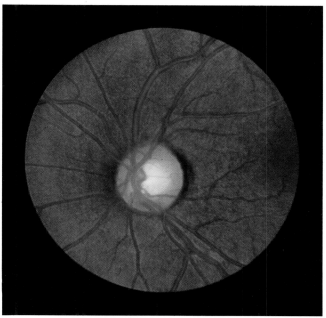

Fig. 8C
A normal fundus in an oriental, illustrating a racial variation in fundus background color. The background is vaguely stippled.

Fig. 9
Glaucomatous optic atrophy. Note the blue-white disc with the white center denoting the lamina cribrosa. The vessels are pushed nasally and do not cross the disc to exit, but go around the rim. They are bent as they leave the disc. A "halo" or white atrophic rim around the disc (especially on the temporal aspect) makes the nerve head look larger than it is.

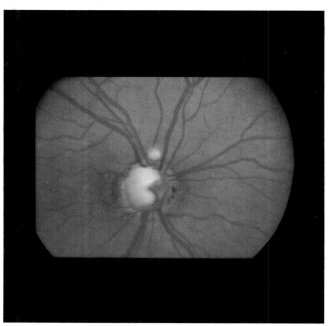

15

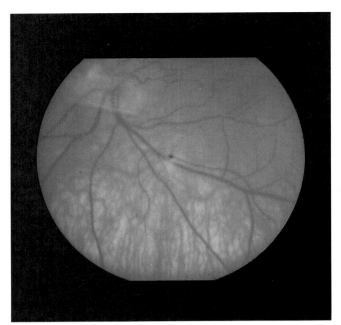

Fig. 10A
The upper quadrant of this retina gives the illusion of anastamotic vessels. This occurs because one sees several layers of superimposed choroidal vessels in the blonde fundus. There is a sharply demarcated veil covering the superior papillary vessels. The veil has an absolutely straight top line and consists of persistent glial tissue.

ally exiting vessels. At the same time the whole bank of central vessels is pushed nasally on the disc, rather than occupying the central area.

Occasionally the round or slightly oval disc appears to have a peculiar shape, as a half moon appearance due to an oblique entrance of the nerve or actual partial coloboma. A coloboma of the disc is an actual absence of part of the disc or a seeming absence due to an oblique entrance of the nerve. We may see cellophane-like white material on the disc, usually cuffing vessels, this is persistent glial tissue. Also visible may be a situs inversus of the disc or of the vessels, which in a right eye would exit at one and five o'clock, then sweep temporally to the temporal retina. When situs inversus is marked, vision is often decreased.

If one disc is yellower or whiter than the other the former should be considered atrophic. This lattter

Fig. 10B
Situs inversus of the vessels on the disc—with the vessels going vertically or nasally before swinging temporally. Visible is a white conus about the disc and a thin choroid, allowing the blotchy white of the sclera to come through.

Fig. 10C
Situs inversus of disc—an obviously inverse or twisted entrance of the optic nerve, with a large chorio-vaginal vein deep to the retinal vessels and a typical coloboma of the choroid below.

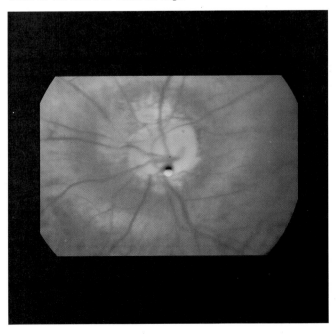

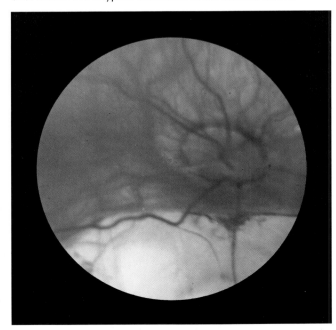

observation may be the first clue to pressure on one optic nerve or to pressure by a chiasmal lesion (usually tumor). Chiasmal tumors usually press one side initially, and cause optic atrophy. Tumors behind the chiasm tend to cause papilledema or swelling of the optic disc by occluding the various foramina through which the cerebrospinal fluid circulates. Normally, the optic discs are not sharply delineated or outlined, in the sense that the nasal margin usually appears slightly blurred, but can be focused with the ophthalmoscope. This is because the largest number of nerve fibers is crowded into the relatively smaller nasal portion of the disc. At the same time the largest temporal portion of the disc contains the relatively smallest number of fibers and therefore appears slightly paler than the rest of the disc. If the disc becomes edematous this will be recognized first nasally, above and below, and later temporally. In a full blown papilledema, whether from optic neuritis or increased intracranial pressure, the disc is so blurred that it cannot be focussed clearly and the vessels, especially the veins, will be engorged. There may be accompanying hemorrhages and transudates which spill over to the adjacent retina. The retina may also become edematous, causing it to appear opaque, striated and grayish in color. A unilateral papilledema, due to increased intracranial pressure, is uncommon. Papilledema per se will not cause decreased vision unless there is visible hemorrhage, transudate or edema of the macula. A unilateral papilledema (also called "choked disc") is most commonly due to optic neuritis, which is often accompanied by decreased vision, even when the adjacent retina appears normal, in contrast to the true papilledema.

During the early stages of embryonic life a blood vessel system arises from the optic nerve running from the disc to the back of the lens, and enmeshing the latter. This system is known as the tunica vasculosa lentis, and is of value only for the ophthalmoscopic residua which may later be visible. Briefly, these vessels go forward from the nasal part of the disc forming a vitreous channel (Cloquet's canal), nourish the lens and then atrophy. If the atrophic process is complete, no residua remain to be seen. If it is incomplete, one or more of the following can be seen. Most commonly seen with the slit lamp is a corkscrew-like thread hanging from the back of the lens; a persistent hyaloid vessel. Rarely seen is a dark vessel emanating from the nasal part of the disc and going forward in the hyaloid or Cloquet's canal, or more commonly (though still infrequent) it may hang down from the nasal part of the disc. The most common remnant is the glial scaffolding of the tunica which remains as a cellophane-like membrane surrounding or "cuffing" some vessels on the disc. At

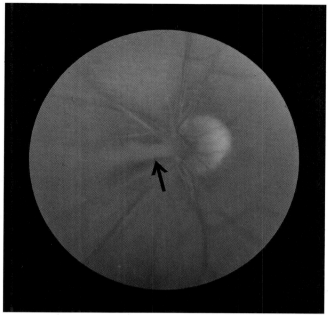

Fig. 11A
The arrow points at a horizontal, gray mass, about four times the width of a retinal vessel, coming off from the nasal part of the nerve head. This is Cloquet's canal, filled with exudative products of a posterior uveitis.

Fig. 11B
Almost two-thirds of this disc appears to be a hazy yellow. This area is a glial tissue mass projecting out into the vitreous and therefore, focused incompletely. It represents incomplete atrophy of the fetal Bergmeister's papilla. The black and white dot to the right is a reflex off a camera.

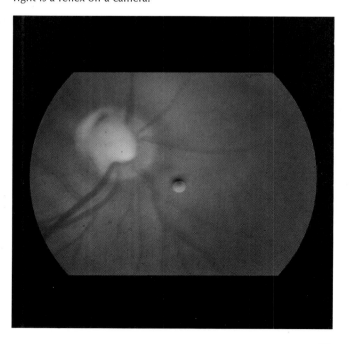

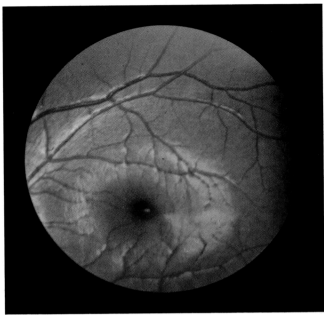

Fig. 12A
Normal macula. Note the avascular dark area of macula, a sharp foveal reflex to one side of the field. It is surrounded by moire silk light reflexes which shift with motion of the ophthalmoscope. The angles formed at the vessel bifurcations are curving rather than angular as is seen in arteriosclerosis.

Fig. 12B
Congenital tortuosity of vessels.

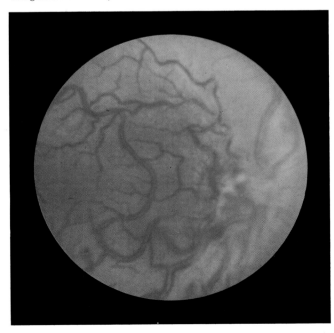

times hemorrhage or transudates will fill the Cloquet's canal, thus outlining it, in front of the disc. At times a considerable amount of the glial scaffolding remains on the disc, resembling a white, glistening cone known as Bergmeister's papilla.

Interpretation of Colors in the Fundus

Color is important when viewing the optic fundus. A knowledge of the normal and abnormal colors and variations of color is useful in making a diagnosis or at least in determining where the problem probably lies. The optic nerve is usually somewhat orange in appearance. Variations from this have already been discussed. The retina is not visible unless it is edematous and therefore is opaquely gray. The normal reddish colored fundus with its dark red veins and lighter, narrower and centrally striped arteries, all seemingly emanating from the disc, obtains its red coloration from the vascular choroid. The latter is the middle of the three coats of the eye and contains three layers of blood vessels, which when visible with the ophthalmoscope give the erroneous impression of crisscrossing in an almost grid-like fashion, in contrast to the retinal vessels which do not crisscross and which always emanate in the disc and bifurcate as they approach the periphery.

The retinal vessels always avoid the macula. The macula is approximately one disc diameters while the fovea is two disc diameters temporally to the disc. "Disc diameters" is a convenient term for measuring the size of a lesion or denoting its site such as "two disc diameters up and temporally to the disc." The disc is approximately 1.5 mm. in diameter. Hence, by reference as an approximate measurement, the size or the location of lesions can be described. In recording or describing lesions, disc diameters becomes convenient for future reference, especially where one is unable to photograph the lesion. One can then describe the lesion as being 1 D.D. (disc diameter) in size and located approximately 2 D.D. up and temporally. This method of measurement facilitates future location of the recorded lesion and deciding whether it has changed size or is now no longer visible.

The choroid is covered with a layer of pigment, as is the retina. If the choroidal pigment is fairly uniform in its distribution, the "retina" will appear uniformly red; but if the choroidal pigment is unevenly distributed, the "retina" will appear streaked or "tigroid" in appearance, and it is referred to as "tessellated." This is most common in dark skinned whites and blacks. In blondes or reddish haired individuals the amount of pigment is decreased, and the fundus (especially in blondes) appears streaked and yellowish. The choroidal vessels may be seen creating the crisscross appearance previously referred to. The observer gets the impression that these vessels are anastamosing, since he is seeing monocularly several crisscrossing layers superimposed upon each other. In a lightly pigmented fundus, such as an extreme blonde or albinic individual one may see the large vortex veins which are not normally ophthalmoscopically visible. Small vessels frequently seen exiting from the temporal side of the disc and going into the macular area are cilioretinal vessels. The macular area is always redder or darker than the rest of the fundus.

Black in the fundus is usually melanin; but may be the result of old hemorrhage with resultant hemosiderin, which is most prominent with the red free light. Occasionally one or several tiny black dots are seen but these are usually insignificant unless occurring in great numbers. In retinitis pigmentosa black spidery corpuscles are seen, most often in the mid-periphery and they are practically always encircling blood vessels, since they occur most commonly in the perivascular spaces; when seen head on with the ophthalmoscope they appear spidery or corpuscular. Retinitis pigmentosa is one of the night blinding diseases. Very deep hemorrhages, as in the choroid, are more apt to appear as dark gray, flat or elevated masses, and may be confused with malignant melanoma of the choroid. Blue or blue-gray, flat areas are apt to be benign nevi of the choroid. When areas of choroiditis heal they tend to become encircled by black (pigment) which may form a black basketwork over the white scar. One may see either (or both) a fine black or a white crescent, (usually) on the temporal side of the disc, and frequently in high degrees of myopia, a white conus or crescent extending around a large part of the disc, temporally. Some fundi appear peppered with fine black or white dustlike particles, which are described as salt and pepper fundi or more precisely as "mostly salt" or "mostly pepper;" the significance of these is not always clear. At times these are abnormal. It is not always possible to account for every dot, spot or "lesion" seen in the fundus, nor may that be necessary. It is the total picture which is important.

White has a number of origins in the fundus. If choroidal tissue is thinned (high myopia) or destroyed (as in choroiditis) the white of the sclera will be seen. In high myopia (approximately −7.00 D or more) this may result in a streaked or brownish pigmented appearance whereas following an inflammatory process as choroiditis there will usually be a dense, black pigment border around the white scar. Transudates, as in hypertension or diabetes or following the resorption of edema or hemorrhage, will leave solid, white areas which appear different ophthalmoscopically than do choroidal scars. Drusen, the small white spots of colloid degeneration of the ret-

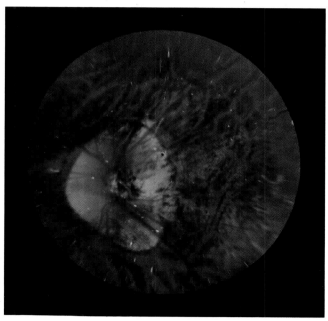

Fig. 13A
Tigroid appearance. Coloboma of part of the disc. Approximately half of the normal orange-colored disc is present. The larger part of the irregular circle is "conus" through which choroidal tissue can be seen. The fundus background is tigroid (tessellated).

Fig. 13B
An albinotic fundus, red retinal vessels and underlying choroidal vessels seen on a virtually white (pigment-free) background.

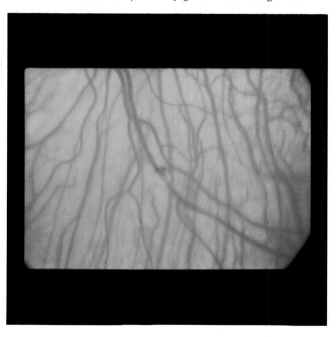

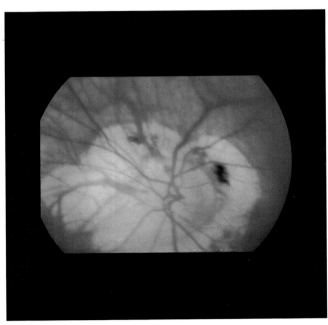

Fig. 14
High myopia with conus. Two features are illustrated: (1) posterior staphyloma and (2) chorio-vaginal veins. The poorly defined circular portion is the disc. The light area surrounding it is naked sclera devoid of choroid (posterior staphyloma). Two types of retinal vessels are visible (a) normal and (b) choroid-vaginal vessels, which are the two thicker vessels with ampulliform dilations near the disc.

Fig. 15
Drusen or colloid degeneration of the retina. Note the fine white dots situated deep to (under) the retinal vessels and interspersed with pigment. The presence of pigment does not necessarily decrease vision.

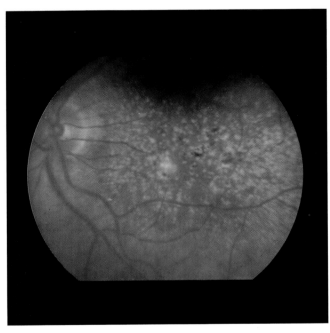

ina, are common in older age groups and are seen as myriads of essentially equal sized white dots underlying the retinal vessels.

The relation of spots to the retinal vessels serves to identify the layer in which the "spots" occur. If lesions encircle or cover the retinal vessels they must be superficial in the retina; if deep to (under) the retinal vessels they must be in the deeper layers of the retina or in the choroid.

Occasionally we see tiny, sharp white dots usually in the midperiphery of the fundus: the histology of these is unclear and they usually are not clinically significant. This is true of many small isolated black or white dots which are seen. When a localized aggregation of white plaques or spots are observed, we tend to relate these to a preceding hemorrhage or collection of edematous fluid, with the spots serving as residua, after the fluid has absorbed. Clinically, many cases have been followed from the original hemorrhage or transudation through the subsequent ophthalmoscopic changes.

At times we see a somewhat stellate white area encircling part of the optic nerve. This white area covers the retinal vessels, tends to be somewhat striate following the nerve fiber distribution, and frays out away from the disc. This is characteristic of congenital medullation of the optic nerve fibers.

In the optic nerve trunk behind the globe, the nerve fibers are covered with a white myelin (medullary) sheath, which disappears when the lamina cribrosa is reached. At times this persists on the visible portion of the disc, as medullated nerve fibers. Since the opaque medullated fibers cover the retina, that portion is "blind," so that the blind spot covered by an optic disc with its extended area of medullation casts a larger than normal blind spot reflecting the ophthalmoscopic picture. Medullated fibers elsewhere similarly create a "scotoma" or blind spot in the visual field. Rarely, the area of medullation will not be at the disc margin, but farther away. Here it will present the same white, striate appearance which outlines the known course of the retinal nerve fibers in this particular site. In the macular area white spots often tend to form circular aggregations.

Certain terms have become synonymous in referring to white spots which are seen with the ophthalmoscope; these are "exudates" and "transudates" or "spots." These may be tiny or may seem to coalesce forming larger areas. They may be "soft" or difficult or impossible to focus sharply because they still contain fluid, or may be "hard" well demarcated and easy to focus. The soft transudates often seen in hypertension are referred to as "cotton-wool" spots. Similar spots are seen in sepsis and in lupus erythematosus. The spots or transudates of diabetes mellitus contain lipoid material and look waxy. Often here as well as in other conditions, cholesterinization occurs and some of the spots become glistening and golden in appearance. The small white spots deep to the retinal vessels, called "drusen" or "colloid degeneration" of the retina, are generally found in older eyes (but may occur in the young) and are due to excrescences on the glass membrane of the choroid. At times there may be associated macular pigmentation and decreased vision.

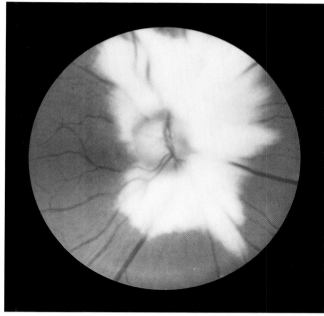

Fig. 16
Persistent medullation of the optic nerve. The optic nerve is engulfed in a sea of white covering the retinal vessels. The white, medullated area feathers out in following the normal course of the retinal nerve fibers.

Fig. 17
Persistent medullation in the retina (away from and not associated with medullation near the disc). The white nerve fibers follow or outline the known course of the retinal nerve fibers.

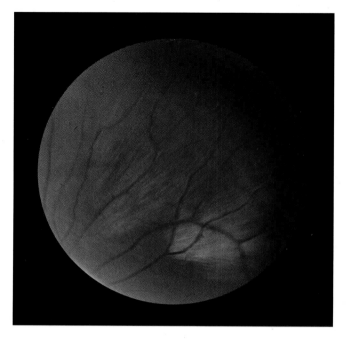

Fig. 18
Macular star and cotton wool spots–the soft, white spots and hard exudates denoted by the sharply demarcated white linear spots.

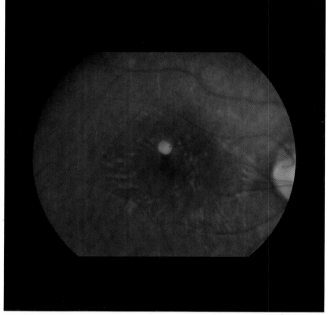

21

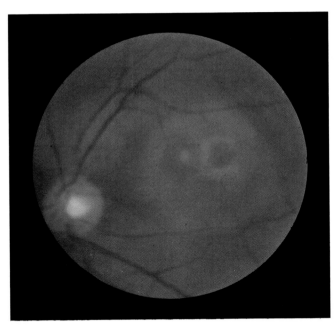

Fig. 19
Macular edema due to an underlying deep choroidal hemorrhage. Neoplasm and intraretinal helminth must be suspected.

When the retina becomes enamatous the fluid forces the nerve fibers apart and renders them more easily visible. When the fluid becomes albuminous the retina then becomes more opaque and grayer in appearance. When the fluid recedes, leaving behind its various constituents, as albumin, fibrin, etc., these latter may be visible as white spots or lines. The macula resembles a table cloth held down in the center by an object (fovea). When its edematous fluid recedes, it looks as though the table cloth had been thrown into folds radiating away from the fixing object (the fovea), so that lines radiate from a central area creating the picture called the "macular star" (Fig. 18). If these solid constituents absorb, the "star" disappears.

Hemorrhages are red when recent, and black or white when old and partially absorbed. They take their shapes from the structures within which they lie and are molded. Hemorrhages in the nerve fiber layer are striated or flame-shaped, tending to be long and narrow. When they are in the middle layers of the retina, they are rounder or bullet-shaped. If preretinal, they assume a flat topped, fluid level, appearance. Deep to the retina, in the choroid, they look like dark gray masses, and may be so dense as to elevate the overlying structures in a tumorlike fashion. In this latter event the overlying retinal vessels will be elevated and present a convexity towards the examiner. The hemorrhages of leukemia tend to have a white center, due to the mode of clearing. This is more commonly seen in adult leukemia than in children. Hemorrhages do not normally occur in the eye and therefore, when seen, must have some significance, even though this may not be readily apparent. Hemorrhages which seem to hang from the disc margin tend to occur from blood dyscrasias or even carcinoma at some distant site in the body. Blood tends to become absorbed, or broken up into several areas (or masses) and the gray areas become smaller or disappear or leave residual white and black spots. Choroidal tumors, in contrast to deep hemorrhages, are usually single and grow slowly. Hemorrhage may occur into or on a tumor, producing more rapid expansion followed by a later decrease in size as absorption takes place. Large hemorrhages in the macular area are often replaced by fibrosis, presenting a yellow, tumorlike mass termed "disciform degeneration of the macula." Aneurysms are seen as single or grapelike collections of tiny red, round dots near blood vessels, and are best visualized when red-free light is employed.

Arterial occlusions tend to be bloodless, with the deprived area becoming edematous. The infarcted area of edema often points at the occluded vessel. Venous occlusions are bloody, with many hemorrhages and transudates. When the central artery of

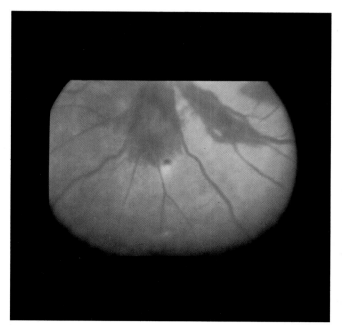

Fig. 20
Myelogenous leukemia in an adult, with large boat-shaped hemorrhages (white center) hanging from the optic nerve (not visible).

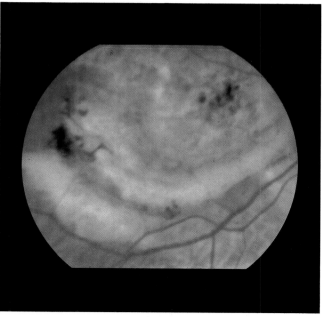

Fig. 21B
Pseudotumor of the retina and choroid following deep choroidal and retinal hemorrhages as in Fig. 19. This lesion is often called a Kuhnt-Junius degeneration or disciform degeneration of the macula.

Fig. 21A
Same patient as Fig. 19—ten weeks later. Note macular edema and transudates.

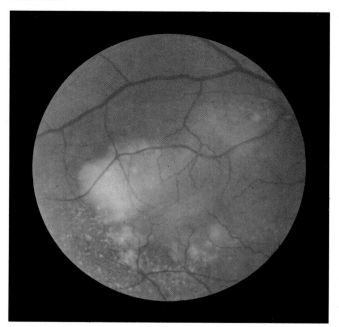

Fig. 22
Occlusion of the central retinal artery with narrowed vessels, retinal edema and cherry-red spot. There is a tiny striate hemorrhage off the disc on the side of the cherry-red spot.

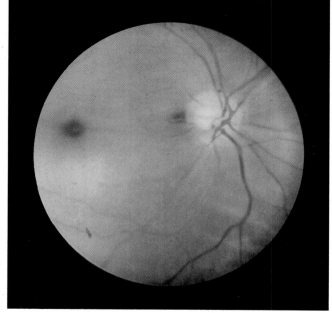

the retina is occluded, the entire retina appears edematous and gray for some days, until canalization of the vessel or collateralization occurs. However, the retina in the macular area is thinner than elsewhere and contains no blood vessels; in fact, the fovea is even thinner. Hence, the relatively thicker retina becomes opaquely gray or white, and the thinner foveal-macular area permits the normal red of the choroid to be seen. The normal red macula seems more brilliant red in contrast to the surrounding opaque retina, thus giving us the "cherry-red spot" of central retinal (or rarely cilioretinal artery to the macula) occlusion. This same situation occurs when lipoid or other material is deposited in the retina as in Tay-Sachs disease, or with a retinal vessel spasm with resulting edema in quinine poisoning. The macula is not redder, the rest of the fundus is whiter. Similarly, in a retinal detachment, when the retina is torn, the brilliant red of the choroid is seen, giving us the red appearance of the "tear" or "break" in the retina.

Other Ophthalmoscopic Clues
The macular area is approximately 3 mm. (2 D.D.) in diameter, subtending approximately 12 degrees of the visual field. The fovea, or center of the macula, is the site of the sharpest vision, and actually lies not at the exact center of the retina but just below the horizontal meridian. In younger people, the fovea is visible as a sharp bright light in the center of the dark circle of macula. With age, the foveal reflex disappears or becomes less bright. When viewed with the ophthalmoscope the macula appears to be encircled by a bright circular reflex or line. If one shifts the ophthalmoscope he sees that the circle is not a fixed line but rather a shifting light reflex. Lesions do not shift with motion of the ophthalmoscope, but light reflexes do, thus serving as an important differential point between (fixed) lesions and the illusory sensation of a lesion obtained from an irregular light reflex. The fovea is actually a shallow pit in the macula, with the foveal reflex appearing as a lighted point at the bottom of the pit.

As pointed out the macular area is free of blood vessels. This means that in the macula there are no anatomical structures which lie between the cones and the light rays which enter the eye from without. The retina contains both rods (important mostly in dark or night vision and in noting motion) and cones (day vision, color and sharp detail vision). The macular area contains only cones and a yellowish pigment which gives it the full name of macula lutea (yellow spot). The retina contains ten layers of cells, fibers, pigment and membranes, but in the fovea the retina thins down to very little more than large cones, so that there is the least possible obstruction to the visual cones from entering light rays.

The retinal blood vessels cover and hence obstruct the retinal elements lying directly underneath, which is why the average patient being viewed through the ophthalmoscope will comment upon the beautiful stripes or snakes which he sees.* Actually an observant or knowledgeable patient can do rough perimetry upon being asked to do so, when viewed through the ophthalmoscope. This is an event which all of you should deliberately experience. Have someone examine your eyes with the ophthalmoscope and visualize your own retina, noting the golden snake-like retinal vessels, and the large "unvesseled" macular area. If there are any lesions in the macula these will be noted by the patient as opacities in that latter area. Some time ago I had a visual problem and asked an ophthalmologist "to take a look at me." He did so and said that I had a small lesion in the macula. I knew that I did not, because I could "see" my own macular area as he examined me and did not see any dark area (scotoma) within the zone delimited by the retinal vessels above and below it.

When approximate measurements are given, it is assumed that the eye being discussed is emmetropic or normal in size and hence also normal from the refraction point of view. If the eyeball is shorter than normal in its anteroposterior axis it is hyperopic or farsighted and if longer than normal the eye is myopic or nearsighted. The size relationships as seen with the ophthalmoscope are altered somewhat by the refractive state of the eye. Myopia (especially over approximately 7 Diopters) tends to be associated with a higher incidence of abnormalities of development than does hyperopia.

The external (outside of cornea to outside of sclera) anteroposterior or sagital diameter normally (emmetropia) is 24.15 mm., transversely 24.13 and vertically 23.48 mm. Hence, the normal eye, although not a perfect sphere is about 25 mm. in diameter. It weighs about 7.5 gm. and has a volume of about 6.5 cc., with a specific gravity of approximately 1.005.

The optic nerve lies nasally to the center of the globe; with the macula functioning as the perimetric,

---

*When a strong light, as from an ophthalmoscope, comes in obliquely, the shadows of the retinal vessels are cast upon a different set of rods and cones than those directly underneath, and they become visible to, and are seen by, the patient as stripes, etc.

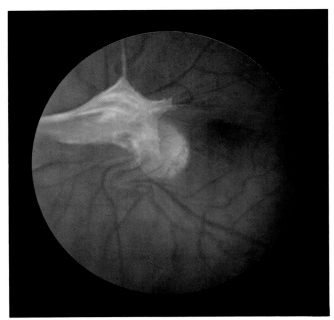

Fig. 23A
A band of fibrous tissue connected to the disc and projecting out in front of it in the vitreous. This followed a severe vitritis, presumably due to Toxocara. The band is exerting traction on the retina in the macular area, throwing the retina into fine traction folds.

Fig. 23B
Wrinkles or stretch lines of the retina radiating about the macula. A leukemic orbital infiltration was suspected.

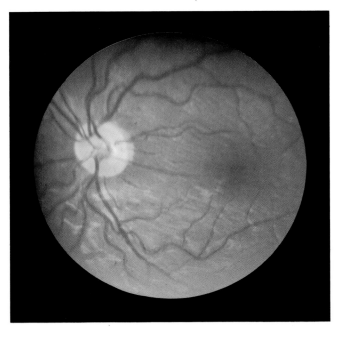

ophthalmoscopic and anatomic center. The nerve lies just below the horizontal meridian and is composed of the retinal nerve fibers. These have approximately one million nerve fibers and do not "see" as do the rods and cones, but merely transmit the visual impulses to the brain, where the actual sensation of seeing occurs in the occipital lobe. The retina is about 0.3 mm. in thickness and the choroid about 0.2 mm.

Ophthalmoscopy
In examining the eye with the ophthalmoscope, the media are examined first by starting with the high-plus lenses and then gradually reducing these until the fundus details become visible. If the examiner has learned how to completely relax his accommodation, the strength of the ophthalmoscope lens used approximates a combination of his refractive error and that of the patient, without taking into account any astigmatic error that either may have. For example, if the examiner is a hyperope of plus 2 and the lens used is plus 4, the patient is also approximately a plus 2. If the examiner has a corrected astigmatic error of significance and finds that the retinal details are distorted without anything in the media causing that distortion, it is safe to assume that the patient has a considerable amount of astigmatism—more than 1 D. Astigmatism simply means that there is a difference in refractive power of the eye horizontally as compared to vertically; due to the fact that the eyeball is not a perfect sphere. Hence, we are all astigmatic, but from a practical viewpoint the important factor is the astigmatism affecting the light rays that reach a focus on the macula. (That which would be observed ophthalmoscopically would, of necessity, be more than the examiner's skill and refraction with glasses could adjust for, and hence would probably be much more than 1 D.) Distortion of one small area of the fundus would not be due to astigmatism.

The wide variation in color of the fundus illustrates the importance of retinal and choroidal pigment. At one extreme one sees dark, blotchy, blackish fundi in negroes and other heavily pigmented people, and almost white fundus backgrounds in albinos at the other extreme. In most instances the fundus color reflects the skin and hair pigmentation. When a blonde fundus is seen in a nonblonde, inquiry will usually reveal that the individual was blonde when younger. The converse may indicate that the hair color came out of a bottle. The background color is never uniform, but rather has a finely granular or stippled appearance, which becomes coarser towards the periphery. Various parts of the same fundus may differ, with one portion being tesselated and another not.

When examining the eyegrounds one should follow a systematic pattern. Examine the optic disc first, then each of the four quadrants which means the upper and lower temporal and the upper and lower nasal areas, and lastly the macula. Once the latter has been flooded with light, the patient becomes photophobic and less cooperative. It often is necessary to hold the patient's eyelids apart, but then he tends to involuntarily resist. It is better if possible for him to stare out in the distance, keeping his own lids apart by conscious effort.

In examining the fundus it is important to move the instrument and to carefully observe the area to each side of the light as well as that portion directly illuminated by the light source. In this manner dark shadows, revealing the presence of hitherto unnoted or unsuspected lesions may be seen. When the light is moved from side to side, vague alterations in the "smoothness" of the fundus can be noted, so that in addition to directly illuminating the lesions we obtain the advantages of indirect and retroillumination.

When a mass is found during fundus examination and a differential diagnosis between a solid mass as a tumor in contrast to a similar appearance due to a hemorrhage or choroiditis becomes important, another mode of using the ophthalmoscope may be most helpful. Remove the ophthalmoscope head and employ the light for transillumination of the globe in a dark room. Instill a drop of topical anesthetic on the eye, and then hold the light against the eye (or the open lids) and move the light around while viewing the transilluminated flowing pupil: If there are no masses visible, the transilluminated pupil will be illuminated fairly evenly. If any masses are present, unless far posterior, they can usually be readily seen. A positive test is important: a negative (failure to visualize) test does not rule out an opaque mass of tumor as compared to a non-opaque mass due to hemorrhage or inflammation, etc.

The retinal light reflexes are more apparent in the young and are said to resemble moire silk. Often, they are so prevalent that the novice examiner is sure that the retina is edematous. At times, and especially near the disc, one can see striations which follow the known course of distribution of the retinal nerve fibers. Three types of lines or folds are seen in the retina, as a rule. One consists of the so-called "macular star", (Fig. 18) which is seen radiating out from the fovea forming its center. Another is the so-called "traction fold" which consists of parallel lines, usually seen in one area and which resemble the sun's rays over a 45-60° angle. This is thought to be due to a pull on the retina by vitreous adhesions, but can also be due to underlying infiltrate (as in leukemia) or a mass pressing from behind the orbit. The last of the commoner (and none of these are common) folds are

Fig. 24
Choroidal wrinkles. Note the concentric curved dark lines, frequently due to an orbital mass pressing on the back of the globe as an orbital metastasis.

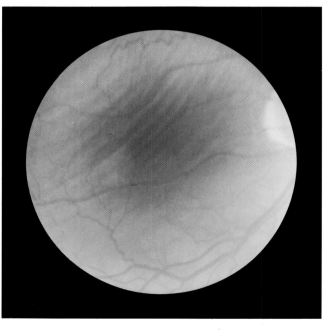

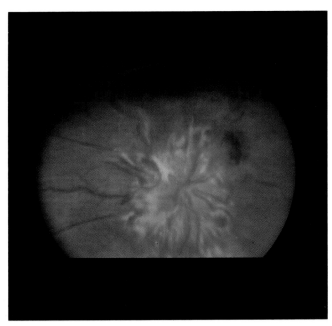

Fig. 25A
Papilledema of 7 disc diopters in a brain tumor. The disc looks like a red and white flower with retinal vessels in the background far behind the disc.

Fig. 25B
A more classical papilledema, with a "choked" disc, tortuous vessels and mild edema of the surrounding retina.

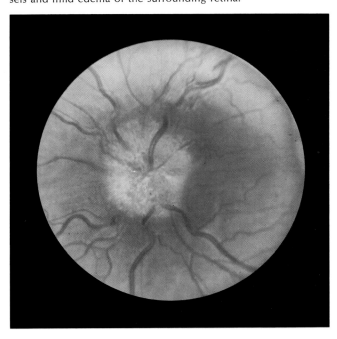

seen as dark, horizontally disposed parallel curved stripes in one quadrant. These are also referred to as "choroidal wrinkles" and are usually due to pressure on the globe by an orbital mass such as a metastatic lesion. At times the source of the folds is not obvious. One patient with traction-type folds in the macula has been under treatment for about 15 years, with no change in either appearance or vision. Similar folds about the macula observed in a leukemic child, have disappeared in a matter of weeks as he responded to therapy, without reappearing as he relapsed.

The Optic Nerve

The opening in the rear of the globe through which the optic nerve exits is bridged by scleral and choroidal tissue, forming a sievelike aperture termed the lamina cribrosa. The optic nerve fibers take on myelin sheathing on the distal (orbital) side of the eye. The ophthalmoscope light reflecting off the myelin sheathing gives the disc its relatively pale coloring. At times the myelin sheathing is seen on the disc and contiguous to it, in the so-called "persistent medullation." The amount of physiologic excavation depends to a certain extent upon the degree of prenatal atrophy of the Bergmeister's papilla, the prenatal support for the vascular tunic to the lens.

One may see no physiologic excavation or one may see all degrees up to a massive excavation apparently taking up most of the disc. In the latter event the physiologic excavation is differentiated from the pathologic excavation caused by the continued increased intraocular pressure of glaucoma because the physiologic excavation always has a rim of normal nerve tissue around it. Advanced glaucomatous atrophy always reaches the very edge of the nerve, creating a sharp border to the latter. This is the textbook description of a glaucomatous excavation. There are two other textbook features: one, that the entire bank of blood vessels is pushed to the nasal side of the disc and secondly, that the blood vessels exiting from the disc temporally bend sharply as they pass over the edge of the pathologically excavated disc and on to the retina. Because the glial and other elements of the center of the disc have atrophied and disappeared there is no tissue framework to support the blood vessels in the center of the disc and these are now located along the disc border. There are several other features of the glaucomatous disc which are important in making the diagnosis. First, it must be borne in mind that the picture which we have just described (Fig. 9) is the picture of an advanced glaucomatous optic atrophy; the end result of the disease. At this stage recognition is easy. The patient will benefit if the diagnosis is made much earlier. It is rarely mentioned that the glaucomatous excavation often takes on a greenish or bluish hue when seen with the ophthalmoscope, in contrast to the white appearance of the excavation in primary optic atrophy due to arterial occlusion, syphilis, trauma to the nerve, etc. Unless a congenital anomaly is present both discs are mirror images of each other. Any obvious difference in the sizes or shapes of the two physiologic excavations means glaucoma in the larger excavation side, unless proved otherwise. This difference in excavation appearance always demands an explanation. When the intraocular pressure is elevated there may be spontaneous pulsation of the artery on the disc. Venous pulsation is a normal event, especially in the young. Arterial pulsation, not transmitted by an underlying, pulsating vein should make the examiner suspicious of glaucoma as it usually results from it. A glaucomatous appearing disc will occasionally be seen in elderly individuals in whom one cannot confirm increased intraocular pressure. This cavernous atrophy is associated with arteriosclerosis, and one can occasionally demonstrate arteriosclerotic carotids pressing on the optic nerve.

The converse of a pathologically excavated disc is an edematous or "choked" disc, which is convex towards the ophthalmoscope in contrast to the concavity presented by a deep excavation. The semantics become somewhat involved and are unimportant if we understand each other. "Papilledema" means an edema of the papilla or optic nerve or optic disc. "Choked disc" means the same thing; the disc appears choked or swollen. Originally these terms were reserved for an edema of the disc due only to increased intracranial pressure. A similar appearance due to an inflamed optic nerve is termed "optic neuritis." These terms implied that one could make the diagnosis with its etiologic implications by means of the ophthalmoscope alone. This is by no means always possible.

There are three chief conditions in which papilledema is noted: (1) increased intracranial pressure due to a growing mass (lesion) within the brain, (2) inflammation of the optic nerve (optic neuritis) and (3) increased intracranial pressure due to hypertension. Optic neuritis is usually unilateral; the other two conditions are bilateral but may be unilateral initially.

The degree of elevation is measured by focusing on the highest point of the swollen disc and then noting the number in the ophthalmoscope aperture. Let us say that this is number 4. One then observes the reading on normally appearing retina which is for example 0. The swelling is 4 diopters. In the emmetropic eye, 3 D. of swelling is equivalent to 1 mm. The observed eye has 1⅓ mm. of edema. The exact amount in mm. is unimportant; the amount in diopters is constant for that eye and is so recorded for future estimation of the progress of the edema.

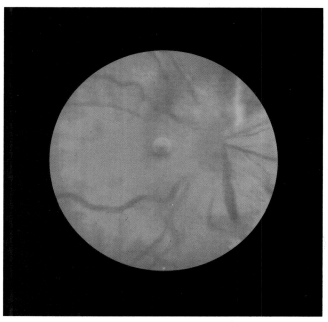

Fig. 25C
Papilledema in an obese woman. There is a choked, blurred disc with retinal vessels converging into it–the veins are tortuous and engorged with one long hemorrhage.

Fig. 25D
Optic neuritis. The disc is slightly blurred, the veins are engorged and the retina is edematous so that the striated retinal nerve fibers are visible. The edema of the disc varies from slight to 3-4 disc diopters of elevation.

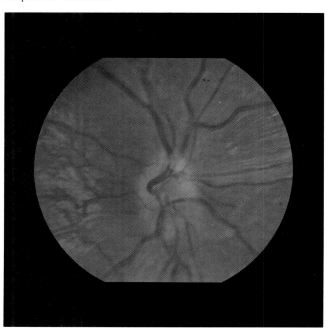

The diagnosis of papilledema may defy the expert when it is early and mild. If one suspects it and is uncertain, that patient should be closely followed, since intracranial pressure tends to increase unless relieved and relief is rarely spontaneous. As edema progresses the excavation becomes filled with transudates. In papilledema, as contrasted to severe pseudopapilledema of hyperopia, the disc appears to be choked but is not and it is difficult to elicit pulsation of veins on the disc. While viewing the fundus through the (preferably dilated) pupil, one presses on the sclera. In the normal eye, the veins now will be seen to pulsate on the disc. In patients with increased intracranial pressure and optic neuritis this is difficult or impossible to elicit. As the edematous disc is larger than normal, it will reflect (or cause) a larger than normal blind spot during perimetry on the tangent screen.

When true swelling of the disc (as differentiated from the pseudo forms which remain constant) decreases, a certain amount of atrophy of the nerve ensues. This atrophy results in a grayish white, dirty appearing disc with residua of the edematous material obscuring the excavation. The edges of the disc remain vaguely blurred.

Optic neuritis (papillitis) is usually unilateral and always associated with marked loss of vision. It is reported to be due to inflammation of the nerve anterior to the lamina cribrosa, in contrast to retrobulbar (behind the eye) neuritis which is said to be due to an inflammatory lesion behind the lamina. Both often occur as a warning sign of multiple sclerosis. Optic neuritis is visible as a swollen nerve, distended veins, many transudates and hemorrhages, possibly some retinal edema, marked loss of vision and field loss. There may also be some pain on motion of the eye. Retrobulbar neuritis, however, shows a marked loss of vision and visual field and little or no ophthalmoscopic changes in the nerve head but there is pain on motion of the globe. To quote Parsons' old dictum "neither the patient nor the doctor sees anything." The pain on motion arises out of the fact that the circle of Zinn from which the four rectus muscles take their origin, encircles the nerve near the site of inflammation, and is irritated by it. The nerve head may or may not appear hyperemic. This is usually difficult to note with certainty and is not especially important in the diagnosis.

On rare occasions the Foster Kennedy syndrome may be seen, with papilledema on one side and optic atrophy on the other. This is due to a tumor of the olfactory lobe or underside of the frontal lobe pressing on one nerve causing it to atrophy. There will be a unilateral loss of sense of smell on this side. An atrophic nerve does not become edematous.

When hypertension is the cause of the nerve edema other ophthalmoscopic (and systemic) signs of hypertension may be found, including marked vessel changes. Occasionally a patient with papilledema will have both hypertension and brain tumor. If the expanding brain lesion, be it tumor, abscess or aneurysm causes other localizing or diagnostic neurologic signs, the diagnosis is facilitated. The chief point is that the ophthalmoscope alone is rarely sufficient as the sole means of diagnosis.

The Retinal Vessels

The retinal vessels are very important in the routine fundus examination, principally because they are so easy to study, because they are involved so often in systemic disease, and because we know so little about the ophthalmoscopic diagnosis of choroidal vessel disease. The retinal vessels exit from (in the case of the artery) and enter into (in the case of the vein) the optic disc. The principal vessels are the central artery and vein of the retina. These both bifurcate to form a superior and inferior papillary vessel, which in turn divides to form the temporal and nasal branches supplying the four quadrants. The vessels continue to bifurcate towards the periphery and do not anastamose. Since the arterial branches lose their muscle fibers and elastic lamina on the retinal side of the lamina cribrosa, they are arterioles rather than true arteries. The retinal vessels have central reflex stripes on their surfaces, which are much more marked in the case of the arteries and are due to light reflected from their surfaces. Certain features mark normal vessels but it is difficult to assess a single vessel without reference to its fellow vessels in the sense of discussing caliber, color, etc. The two lines which ophthalmoscopically delineate a specific vessel are always parallel and deviations are abnormal. The veins are darker and wider than the accompanying arteries with an approximate 3:2 ratio. The retinal vessels are graceful in their course throughout the fundus, exhibiting gently curving bifurcations. There may be a congenital tortuosity of the vessels continually curving in their course. Curving bifurcations are emphasized as they differ from the acute angled bifurcations observed in vessel sclerosis and spasm.

As the vessels pass to the retinal periphery the arteries and veins cross each other, the artery usually remaining at one level and the vein passing underneath. The reverse is less common but when it occurs the vein may appear to form a convexity (hump) towards the observer as it crosses the artery. At the sites of crossing a common adventitial sheath is present. These crossings are significant ophthalmoscopically in the detection of vessel disease. Normally, where the artery crosses the vein, the latter may be seen through the crossing artery. The fact that it cannot be seen may be normal, or it may be an early arteriosclerotic sign and its significance may be difficult to interpret as an isolated phenomenon.

Arteriosclerosis may be part of a hypertensive process or may be involutional. During the forties and early fifties it is more apt to be hypertensive, and then in individuals with a family history of hypertension or vascular accidents occurring early in life. Crossings become abnormal and significant when alterations occur in the veins on either side of the arteriovenous (AV) crossing. In arteriosclerosis there will be observable narrowings and alterations in the parallelism of the vessel walls at the AV crossings. At times the vein will appear to be deflected away by the crossing artery; this is not abnormal. But when the veins narrow down, lose their reflex stripes and appear darker on either or both sides of the AV crossing, this is significant in evaluating the hypertensive-arteriosclerotic state. At times the underlying vein will be fuller before it passes under the artery, as though its return circulation is impeded. At times the underlying vein seems to fade away as it narrows down on either side of the artery, forming the so-called Gunn's sign. This is thought to be due to a sclerotic process affecting the common adventitial sheath of the crossing artery and vein. There is insufficient histologic evidence to support this idea but there is considerable clinical evidence for its validity. Another similarly important sign is the Salus' sign which refers to the U-shaped bending away or displacement of the underlying vein as it seems to be trying to get away from the overlying artery.

The caliber of the arteries and veins may be increased or decreased. When the arteries dilate or increase in caliber there is an associated increase in tortuosity of the artery. When the caliber narrows, as in involutionary sclerosis or in arterial spasm, there is a lengthening and straightening in course of the affected artery. When the arteries become more dilated or "fuller" there is an associated increase in the brilliance of the arterial reflex stripe. Narrowing may affect all of the arteries, some of them or only part of one vessel. In narrowing, the artery becomes less visible and less brilliant in appearance. Vessel spasm is often "toxic" in that it may be seen during the toxic phase of hypertension, in eclampsia, in drug intoxication and in the mother before immediate fetal death. The localized narrowings may be spastic or may be due to localized sclerotic changes or to atheromatous plaques (Fig. 53) which may be seen as small white areas "in" the vessel wall. Occasionally a transient white "plaque" may be seen in a vessel wall, only to disappear. These are thought to be due to temporary collections of platelets. These plaques of atheromata or platelets appear to be within the arterial reflex stripe ophthalmoscopically, since we do not have monocular depth perception. If they protrude significantly over the sides of the vessels and cover the vessels then it would be safe to assume that they lie over the vessel and are not part of its walls. By the same token, if the "plaque" could be seen under the vessel, whose walls at that point were transparent, it could be assumed that we were dealing with a retinal lesion which was not part of the overlying vessel.

Three colors are important in describing presumably abnormal arteries: coppery, silver wire and white sheathing. The "copperiness" is seen in the increased highlight of the reflexes of dilated, tortuous arteries in hypertension and vascular disease. The "copperiness" may decrease if the underlying condition responds to therapy. Silver wiring is usually patchy, affecting only one or several branches as a rule. These vessels are narrowed, with pale blood columns and bright, silvery reflex stripes along the vessel axes. This condition is not necessarily associated with hypertension, but is due to a loss of vessel wall transparency due to vessel disease. In "sheathing" the artery appears to be encased during part or all of its course by a white sheath, or the whole artery appears white and nonfunctioning. The latter is illusory, as there is rarely evidence of occlusion of the sheathed vessel. The sheathing may be seen as two white lines on either side of the vessel, partly or completely replacing the arterial walls, on either side of the central reflex stripe or as a white vessel. This may be seen as a rare congenital anomaly in the infant. Most commonly it follows optic neuritis, perivasculitis or vasculitis as in the vasculitis of young adults termed Eales' disease or in periarteritis nodosa or syphilis.

Venous changes may occur which are similar to those already noted in the arteries. Those most commonly seen are in the direction of dilation, tortuosity, caliber variations, sheathing, sluggishness of circulation with edema and hemorrhages, neovascularization, varicosities, loops and aneurysms.

We have noted that narrowing or spasm is common in arteries; the reverse, dilatation, is more common in veins and is associated with increased tortuosity. At times the degree of dilation is enormous and may be generalized as in an occlusion of the central retinal vein or localized as in an occlusion of a branch of the vein.

Sheathing of the veins is most commonly seen in venous obstruction, diabetic retinopathy and Eales's disease. Venous sclerosis is referred to as phlebosclerosis and inflammation as phlebitis. The veins often seem to be patchily sheathed with pigment as in retinitis pigmentosa a night blinding disease where the perivascular pigment rarely involves arteries. In certain blood dyscrasias (leukemia and diabetes mellitus)

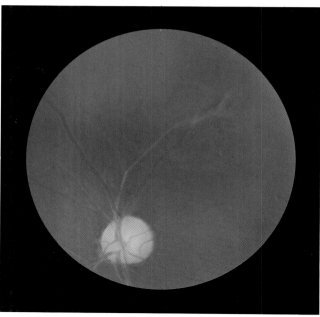

Fig. 26A
Optic atrophy with sheathed vessels. The disc is sharply outlined. This picture is compatible with a post-vasculitis.

Fig. 26B
Venous loop on the disc. A normal variation of the vascular pattern.

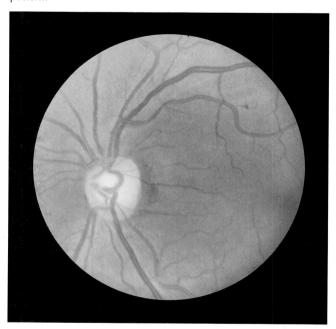

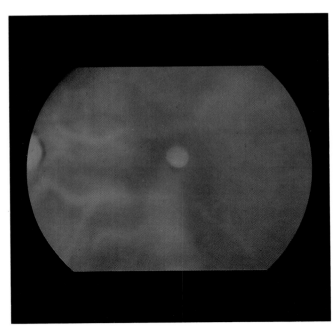

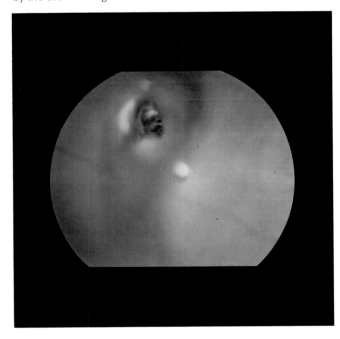

there may be sheathing of the veins with blood which has seeped through the vessel walls by diapedesis. Neovascularization of vessel walls may be seen similarly. At times a collateral circulation may set up in the veins around the site of a venous occlusion, presenting a picture of a box of veins surrounding this site. Varicosities of the veins are occasionally seen in Osler-Rendu disease (familial hereditary telangiectasis). Venous loops in front of the disc may occur as a congenital phenomenon.

Bifurcation of the central vessels into their papillary branches, followed by bifurcation of the papillary vessels, occur within the nerve, on its face or in front of the disc. These various sites of bifurcation account for the variations in the normal appearance of the nerve. If the bifurcation takes place within the nerve, the nerve head will appear to be a mass of vessels. If it takes place out in the vitreous in front of the nerve, then one has the impression that his view of the disc is obscured by vessels. The important factor is to view the nerve head in terms of the presumed site of bifurcation of the central vessels. Occasionally a cilioretinal artery is visible and is so frequent in occurrence that it should be easily identifiable. One or two of these vessels are often seen coming out of the disc, usually on the temporal side, and passing to the macular area. If large they may be the sole source of arterial blood to the macula and may be occluded even though the central artery is not. In this condition there is a central blindness while in the periphery outside of a 10-12 degree perimetric circumference there is normal vision. The cilioretinal arteries come from the vascular circle of Zinn as distinguished from the macular circle of Zinn.

A rarer sight is that of an opticociliary vein. This is a large vein which seems to come out on the disc and then go right back forming a small loop on the surface of the disc. This is not to be confused with the many fine calibered nutrient vessels seen on the disc surface which do not exit onto the retina.

Vitreous
The vitreous is a gel filling up the posterior portion of the eye behind the lens. The vitreous is important ophthalmoscopically because it is frequently the site of opacities which may be considered both normal and abnormal depending upon their appearance and their cause. As a rule the patient who has opacities in the vitreous will complain of seeing spots which he may describe and draw as looking like spiders, flies or threads. True vitreous opacities, as distinguished from a retinal lesion, cause motile spots. When the patient has vitreous opacities he will describe these spots as floating all over but not floating exactly with the motion of the eye, whereas a spot or scotoma

(blind spot) in the visual field, will be seen as a spot which always follows the motion of his eye.

Vitreous opacities may occur normally in myopia and pathologically in old age as a degenerative process or following hemorrhages, due to vascular changes within the eye but more especially in diabetes and hypertension. In arteriosclerosis vascular changes in the eye may result in leakage of blood into the vitreous and certain inflammations producing phlebitis may cause an erosion of a blood vessel with massive bleeding. Trauma may also produce retinal hemorrhages. Inflammations of the eye due to uveitis, and the passage of a nematode into the vitreous, may result in an exudation of cells into the vitreous with massive opacities. In synchysis scintillans, which has been previously mentioned, the condition is characterized by the appearance of numerous gold, glistening particles in the vitreous. These particles are due to various salts of cholesterol and calcium and are rarely noted by the patient. One third of these cases will be found to have a disturbed glucose tolerance test, which is said to be true of this older age group where this condition usually occurs. Vitreous bands follow repeated vitreous hemorrhages as well as occurring as congenital anomalies.

Myopia

Myopia consists essentially of two types; (1) normal myopia, in which the eyeball is longer than normal and for which the patient requires concave lenses in order to see at a distance, (2) the pathologic higher degree of myopia. It is difficult to define the term "high myopia" exactly. When one achieves a myopia of more than approximately −7 diopters, he may be said to have high myopia, (Fig. 14) and somewhere in this area the unusual changes begin to become apparent, due to excessive stretching and elongation of the eyeball with its effect on the vitreous, retina and choroid. The myopic changes affect the entire eye but, more especially, the vitreous, the region of the optic nerve, and the macula. These changes are due to an oblique entrance of the optic nerve into the sclera so that a super traction occurs on the nasal side of the disc with the retina seeming to be pulled up onto the disc, whereas, temporally there is a white or white-yellow crescent (conus) around the optic nerve. When this stretching of the eyeball becomes too great for the retina and choroid to withstand, the choroid becomes thinned and a large, whitish, yellow area of circumpapillary atrophy is seen, so that it is difficult at times to appreciate where the optic nerve border ends and the area of choroidal atrophy begins. As stated before, when one sees large, white yellowish areas in the fundus, he may be looking at sclera, which means that the choroid has either completely or incompletely atrophied. During incomplete atro-

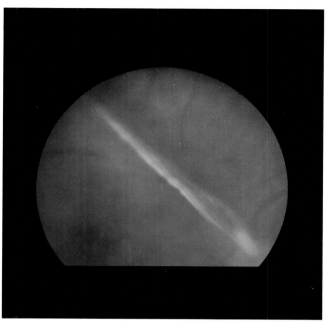

Fig. 28
Congenital retinal fold, extending from the disc into the periphery in the vitreous. This is primary persistent hyperplastic vitreous.

Fig. 29
An area of posterior staphyloma is seen on the left side of the picture with two oval areas on the right. The latter are areas of stretching and atrophy of the choroid in high myopia. They are crossed by retinal vessels.

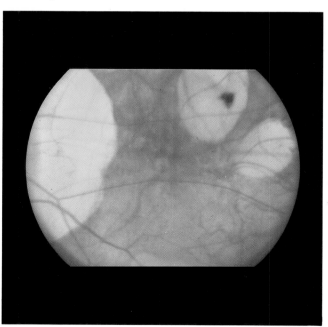

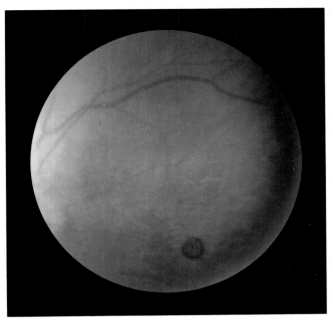

Fig. 30
Fuchs' black dot—a sharply demarcated black dot caused by a hemorrhage into the fovea in high myopia.

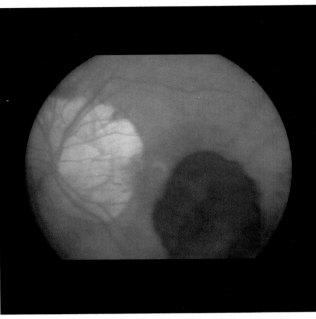

Fig. 32
Huge macular hemorrhage in a high myopia—observe the black hemorrhage and the white conus on the temporal side of the disc.

Fig. 31
A dense pigment spot in the fovea, surrounded by an area of depigmentation. Results from hemorrhage into the foveal area with slow absorption. Note the "cracks" (streaks) in the macula, an aftermath of a Fuchs' dot.

Fig. 33
Similar to Fig. 32 showing a white area of clearing and red residual blood.

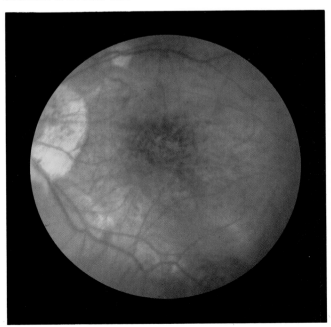

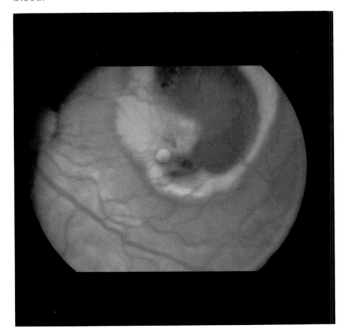

phy we see choroidal vessels which look like flat red bands in the white area. The stretching produces cracks and even areas of atrophy in the macula. At times a small red or black spot resulting from a hemorrhage in the fovea may be seen. This obviously abolishes central vision. This spot is referred to as a "Fuch's dot." The rest of the fundus may exhibit yellowish areas of disseminated atrophy. At times, the retina will tear so that the brilliant red of the choroid will show through as a red triangular or crescentic-shaped area. This is a retinal tear, where one is looking not at the retina but at the choroid which is exposed by the torn retina above it. The vitreous in myopia may become very liquid so that with the slit-lamp one can see the entire vitreous body moving rapidly with motion of the eye.

Hyperopia has few abnormalities associated with it unless it is extremely excessive in the neighborhood of plus 10 or 12 diopters. This is a rare event but occurs when the lens is removed and the eye becomes aphakic. Essentially the change seen in hyperopia of approximately +5 diopters or more is pseudoneuritis.

Diseases of the Optic Nerve
Many diseases affect the optic nerve either primarily, or secondarily. Changes in the retina causing atrophy of the retinal nerve fibers produce changes in the optic nerve itself.

Optic Atrophy
Inflammatory or degenerative changes of the retina, trauma to the optic nerve and occlusions of the central retinal vessels or of their branches will cause patchy or complete atrophy of the optic nerve. Atrophy of the optic nerve indicates a concomitant loss of the nutrient blood vessels on the disc which previously showed a white or white-yellow appearance ophthalmoscopically. We often refer to optic atrophy as either primary or secondary. It is primary if the condition producing the atrophy was primarily within the optic nerve itself. This usually means either trauma to the optic nerve or occlusion of the central retinal artery. Primary optic atrophy (usually means vascular atrophy) presents a white disc with fairly sharp edges in which the physiological excavation is visible with the silvery dots of the lamina cribrosa seen in its floor. There has been excessive atrophy of glial tissue baring the excavation further. If the atrophy is due to occlusion of one artery, then only that part of the disc from which that artery emanates, will be white. In glaucomatous atrophy, there will be a bluish white disc with sharp edges and a large excavation. When optic atrophy follows degeneration of the macula, there may be a marked pallor of the temporal part of the disc. If the optic atrophy is secondary to some

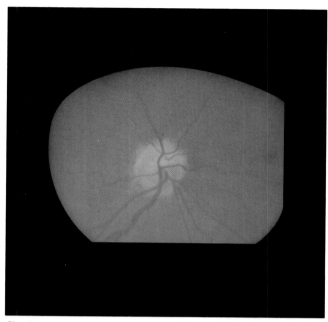

Fig. 34
Hemi-atrophy of the optic nerve, due to closure of a papillary artery. The upper half of the disc is paler than the lower with the arteries all but nonexistent.

Fig. 35
Primary optic atrophy with a white, sharply outlined nerve head. This usually follows vascular (arterial) occlusion.

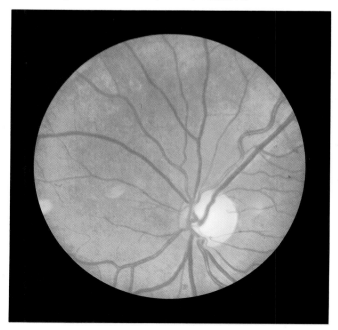

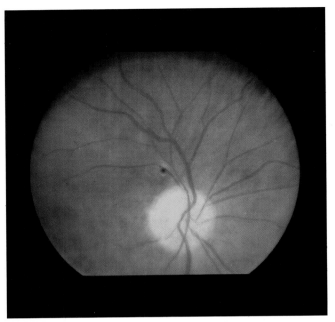

Fig. 36
Secondary optic atrophy with blurred papilla following nerve inflammation. The retinal arteries are much narrower than the veins.

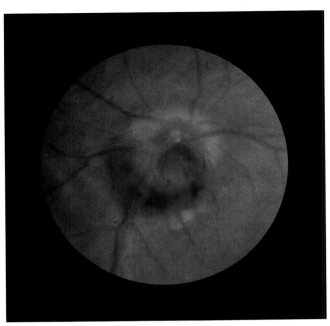

Fig. 37B
Melanocytoma of the disc, a pigmented cyst lying on the nerve head.

Fig. 37A
Grayish disc surrounded by a white ring of tissue. The vessels climb down off the disc over the white ring. This rare tumor of the optic nerve compresses the nerve.

Fig. 37C
Melanocytoma of the optic nerve seen as clumps of pigment obscuring the nerve head.

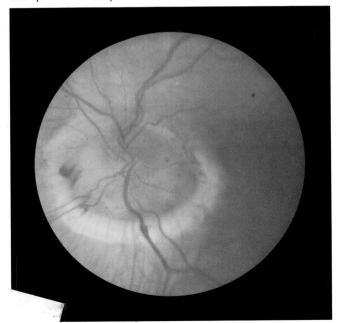

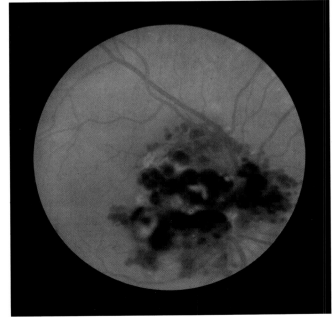

inflammation of the nerve, a secondary atrophy ensues. This is characterized by a dirty yellow disc with blurred borders in which the physiological excavation has been completely filled in with exudative products and therefore is not visible. In both of these situations, fine, nutrient blood vessels which are commonly seen on the disc, will be completely or partially absent. One cannot always make a diagnosis of the etiology of the optic atrophy from the appearance of the disc but he can usually divide it either into a primary or secondary form and then work backward to the unknown etiology from that point. When inflammation of the disc has been present some of the blood vessels coming off the disc may remain sheathed. Brain tumor may cause either papilledema when there has been increased intercranial pressure or optic atrophy when the tumor is in the region of the chiasm. In the latter case, the optic atrophy will be a descending type, affecting one side before the other. It takes about eight weeks after the pressure on the optic nerve or chiasm has started to become pathologic before the atrophy can be seen.

Primary nerve tumors are rare. Some will be noted under phakomatosis.

Retinopathies

The term "retinopathy" refers to any condition which affects the retina, degenerative, vascular, traumatic or inflammatory. Many retinopathies are a reflection of systemic disease elsewhere in the body, such as hypertension, diabetes, leukemia, septicemia, kidney disease, the blood dyscrasias, etc. Theoretically, the term "retinitis" should be reserved for inflammatory conditions of the retina. Those conditions which are reflections of systemic conditions elsewhere will cause changes in the region of the blood vessels, especially in the form of localized edema or white spots which are usually soft and difficult to focus as well as hemorrhages. Where there is true infection within the eye with organisms carried to the retina, there will be true retinal exudates, usually close to the retinal blood vessels. This means that when one examines the fundus systematically, special attention should be paid to the region of the optic nerve, to the blood vessels and to the macula since these are the most important areas ophthalmoscopically. Occasionally seen is what appears to be sclerosis of the choroidal vessels, visible as a meshwork of white, irregular lines.

Retinal Hemorrhages

Retinal hemorrhages may occur from any one of a number of causes but especially in hypertension, arteriosclerosis, myopia, phlebitis, occlusion of a branch or all of the central retinal vein, in the blood

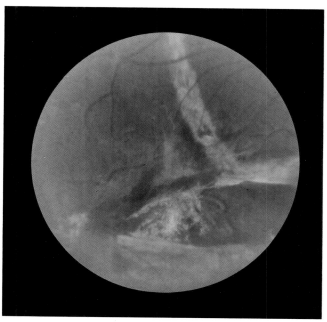

Fig. 38
Cysticercosis. This is a destructive retinopathy following intraocular death of the organism. The bands are a form of retinitis proliferans (common in diabetes).

Fig. 39
Soft cotton-wool spots in a 24-year-old male with chronic nephritis. The A-V ratio is about 1:3.

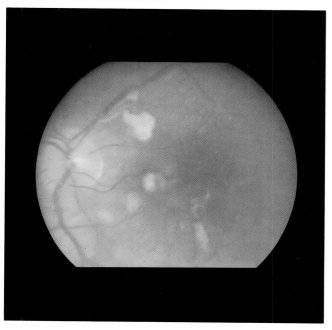

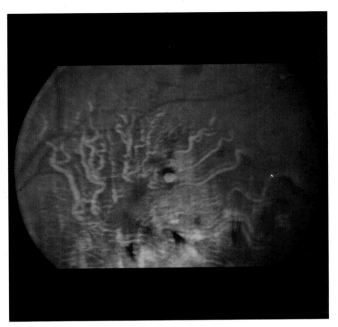

Fig. 40
Choroidal sclerosis. The white (sclerotic) vessels lie deep to the retinal vessels.

dyscrasias and in metabolic diseases, especially diabetes as well as after trauma. If the hemorrhage is large, it may break through the limiting membrane of retina and into the vitreous. As there are no vitreous blood vessels, there cannot be a vitreous hemorrhage per se. At times one may see a lesion at a retinal blood vessel causing the hemorrhage; but as a rule the exact area of bleeding is not easy to find. It is not the purpose of this book to discuss treatment. However, when we find the site of recurring hemorrhages, as in diabetes, it may be possible to photocoagulate the site of the bleeding and prevent future episodes. When there is considerable blood in the vitreous, it becomes impossible to make out good retinal detail.

Vessel Occlusions
Two of the most devastating vascular accidents which can occur within the eye are occlusion of the central retinal artery or one of its branches and occlusion of the central retinal vein or one of its branches.

Occlusion of the Retinal Arteries
A retinal blood vessel may be occluded by an embolus, a thrombus or a local or diffuse spasm. It is not always possible to tell just what is causing the occlusion. Arterial occlusions are differentiated from venous occlusions by the fact that the arterial occlusions are bloodless, whereas the venous occlusions are

Fig. 41
Retinal hemorrhage with an overlying cilioretinal artery. The arteries are straight and narrow, typical of Grade 1 vessel change.

Fig. 42
Bright plaque embolus in a vessel—standing out like a tiny golden dot following a carotid thrombus with endarterectomy.

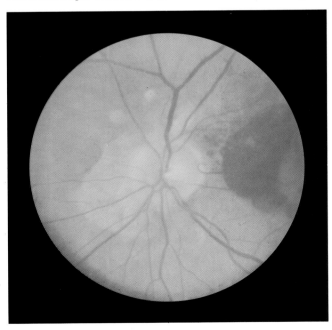

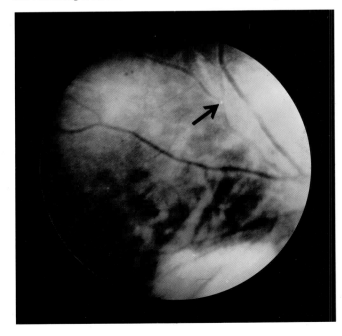

bloody, and if the venous occlusion is in only one branch just that quadrant of the retina drained by that vein will be covered with blood. However, if that quadrant is one of the superior quadrants, some of the blood may seep down below the area normally affected by that vein, so that an area larger than a single quadrant of hemorrhage will be observed.

In arterial occlusion there will be massive edema of the area involved so that the retina becomes opaque. We have already discussed the mechanism of the "cherry-red spot." Hence, when an occlusion of the artery affects either the central artery or cilioretinal artery to the macula, the cherry-red spot of choroid will be seen through the surrounding opaque retina and will give the characteristic appearance seen in occlusion of the central artery, e.g., Tay-Sachs disease, quinine poisoning, as well as other conditions causing the macular area to become opaque. The ophthalmoscopic appearance varies depending upon the time lapse after the occlusion. During the initial days the disc margins will be blurred, the retina gray white, and the cherry-red spot present. The involved arteries will be so attenuated as to be hardly visible. After approximately a week, the edema begins to subside and the cherry-red spot disappears. The arteries become fuller and the disc begins to atrophy. The normal moire silk retinal reflexes will disappear in the areas of atrophy. If the central retinal artery is occluded,

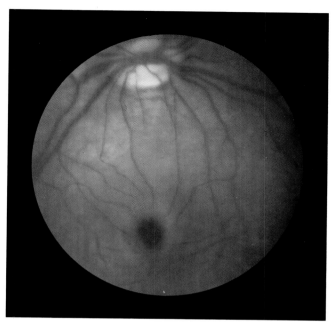

Fig. 43B
Tay-Sachs disease—cherry-red spot. The gray surrounding the cherry-red spot is due to the degeneration and heaping of the ganglion cells.

Fig. 43A
Occlusion of the central retinal artery with perimacular edema, cherry-red spot and the fragmented blood column described as "box-carring" or "trucking."

Fig. 44
Occlusion of a branch of the central retinal artery. Note the large hemorrhage off the disc.

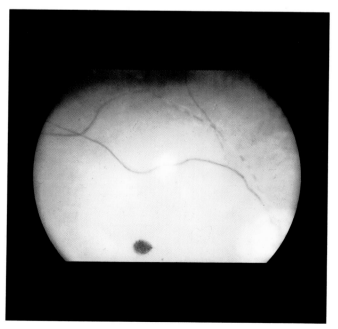

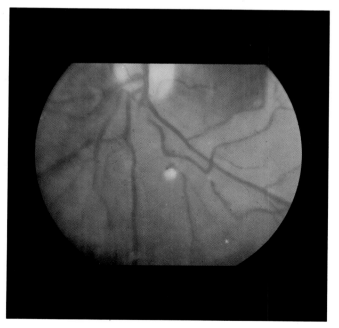

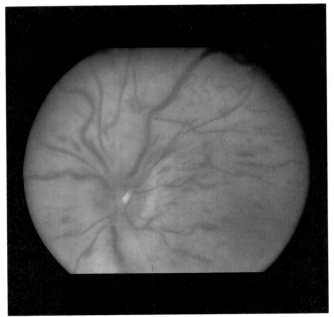

Fig. 45
Occlusion of the central retinal vein. All of the veins are engorged and there are hemorrhages and transudates in all retinal quadrants. Most occlusions are more nearly complete, so that more hemorrhages and transudates are present. The disc is not edematous but is difficult to visualize through the hemorrhages and overlying engorged vessels.

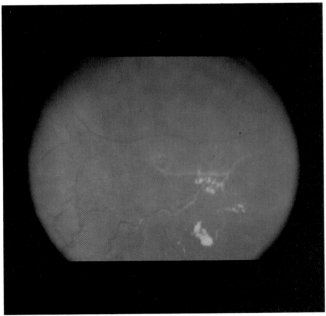

Fig. 47A
Old occlusion of a branch of the central vein. The occluded (sheathed) veins and the red unoccluded veins come together to form a box-like anastamosis or collateral circulation.

Fig. 46
Occlusion of the superior papillary vein. The veins in the field are engorged and the hemorrhages and transudates are confined to one-half the retina.

Fig. 47B
Sheathing of a vein following a branch occlusion. Note the "white vessels" and residual bullet-shaped hemorrhages.

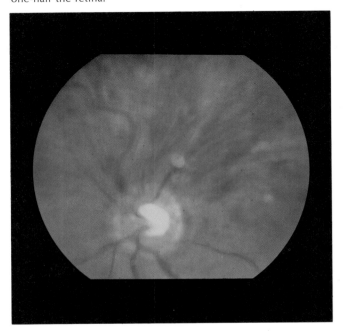

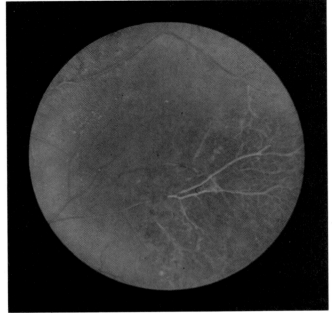

the entire fundus loses its lively reflexes. At the present time there is no known effective treatment for occlusion of a retinal artery. One attempts to decompress the eye by paracentesis of the anterior chamber with a simultaneous whiff of amyl nitrate, or other retinal vasodilators, which are usually ineffective.

Venous Occlusions

If the central retinal vein is occluded, one sees a markedly swollen disc. The veins are hyper-dilated and thrown into a tortuous pattern. The entire fundus is covered with hemorrhages, white yellowish transudates and edema. The arterioles are characteristically attenuated and vision will be virtually absent. At times, there may be incomplete occlusion of the central vein, with an appearance similar to that just described in the face of fairly good vision. These are the patients who respond virtually to any treatment because the occlusion has been incomplete and will eventually take care of itself. On rare occasions, the patient will form a collateral circulation which will spontaneously take care of the occluded vein. Secondary glaucoma may occur as a later complication of central retinal vein occlusion. Occlusion of a branch of the central vein creates a similar picture with the retinopathy limited to a quadrant. The occluded vessels may become sheathed with secondary optic atrophy ensuing. The treatment for occlusion of the central retinal vein or its branches has been anticoagulants. Recently, the use of dextran 40 has been advocated and apparently seems to be of value.

The Retina in Systemic Disease

Hypertension

Hypertension is probably one of the two most important systemic diseases with which our reader will be involved when he views the fundus; the other is diabetes mellitus. The terms hypertension and arteriosclerosis refer to two separate conditions which often may be associated or arise out of each other. In referring to vascular retinopathies, it is difficult to avoid disassociating the two conditions. There are many classifications of hypertensive retinopathy which simultaneously take into consideration the arteriosclerotic features. It is not our purpose to become involved in semantics; but we shall attempt to point out where the two become intermingled. Most descriptions of hypertensive retinopathy are based on the Keith-Waggoner classification which classifies the fundus from Grade 1 to Grade 4. *Grade 1* may be considered as that in which the arterioles become narrowed and straightened in their course and begin to exhibit sharp or acute angled bifurcations. In *Grade 2* arteriovenous compressions become prominent. Here one notes increased "copperiness" of the central arterial reflex stripes, probably an arteriosclerotic man-

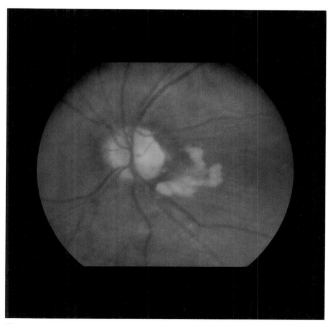

Fig. 48
Patient with congenital heart and Burger's disease presenting a large transudate near the disc, retinal edema, straight retinal arteries and some rather acute angled bifurcations.

Fig. 49
Grade 1 vessel change. An early arterial change, a straightened artery and one obtuse bifurcation.

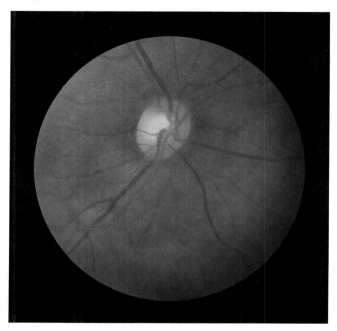

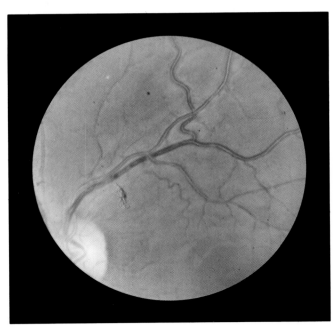

Fig. 50
Grade 2 vessel changes–arteriovenous compression. Where the artery crosses the vein, the vein is hidden by the overlying artery. The vein adjacent to and on the disc side of the crossing seems to be missing–the earliest evidence of true A-V compression.

ifestation. Those veins which cross over arteries are pushed away from the artery, forming a distinct hump; or the underlying veins are deeply compressed by the arteries and seem to disappear on either side of the arteriovenous crossing. On careful observation of the pathologic arteriovenous crossings, the retina may be seen to be endematous, or there may be soft, so-called "cotton-wool spots." One must be careful to differentiate between a pathologic arteriovenous compression and a crossing in which one cannot see the underlying vein. A *Grade 3* retinopathy is one with retinal hemorrhages and transudates present. The hemorrhages are often flame-shaped; they lie in the nerve fiber layer, whereas transudates are usually soft, whitish-yellow areas which are near arteriovenous crossings but may be scattered. It is difficult to state exactly where Grade 2 ends and Grade 3 begins, if only several transudates are present. A *Grade 4* retinopathy is that stage in which papilledema is present. The retinopathy does not necessarily progress from Grade 1 to Grade 4. One may see papilledema in hypertension with few retinal vessel changes. This may be a situation which has come on suddenly because of a marked increase in intracranial pressure. The arteriosclerotic features of the retinal vessels are obviously those affecting the vessels themselves. These may be seen as atheromata or persistent white

Fig. 51A
Grade 3 vessel changes with A-V compression and a hemorrhage at the site of the compression, plus massive cotton-wool (soft) spots. Patient had hypertension of 250/130.

Fig. 51B
Another form of Grade 3 hypertension retinopathy with straight narrow arteries, marked retinal edema outlining the course of the nerve fibers, flame-shaped hemorrhages and cotton-wool spots.

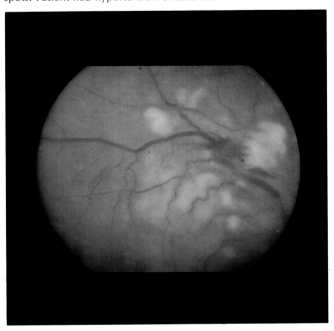

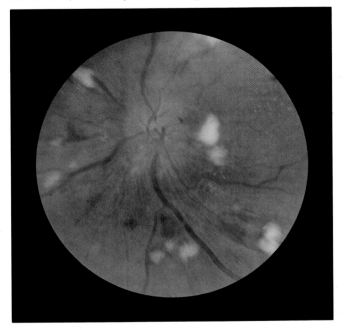

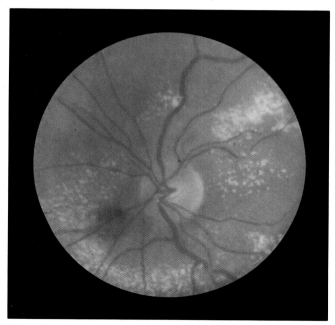

Fig. 51C
Grade 3 hypertensive-arteriosclerotic retinopathy. The arteries are coppery with widening of their reflex stripes. The veins are engorged with one golden plaque overlying a vein on the disc. There is a marked A-V compression in the lower field.

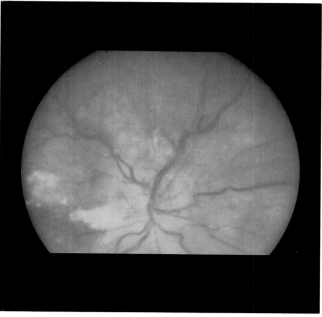

Fig. 52B
Grade 4 changes with edema and obscuration of the disc, marked engorgement and caliber variations of the vessels, marked A-V compressions and transudates.

Fig. 52A
Grade 4 retinopathy in hypertension. The disc is visible, overlaid with edema and transudates.

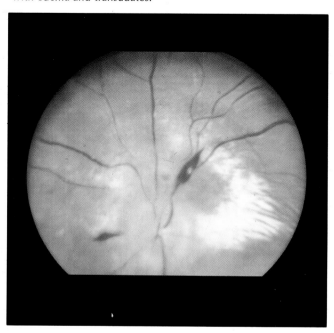

Fig. 52C
Macular star in Grade 4 hypertension, edema of the disc, A-V compressions, with marked transudates forming a star-shaped figure in the macula. There is Salus' sign in the lower field, where the silver wire artery deeply indents and pushes away the underlying vein which forms a U as it is deflected by the artery.

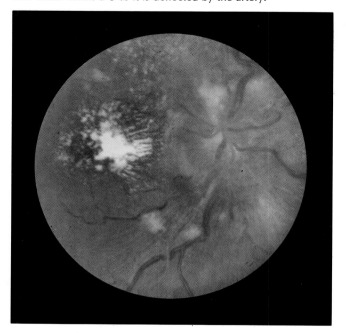

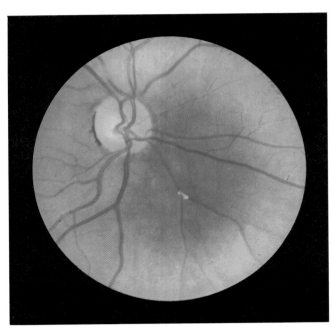

Fig. 53
The white plaque within the bifurcation is probably an atheroma.

Fig. 54
Two of the arteries are coppery and one is silver-wired (sheathed). A corkscrew vessel hanging from the disc represents an old occluded branch.

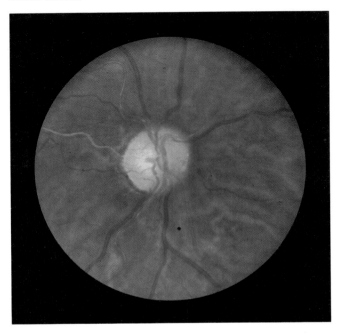

spots in a retinal vessel wall as caliber narrowings, so that the parallelism of the retinal walls is no longer present or in a marked "copperiness" or even a silver wire appearance of the retinal vessels. There may also be hemorrhages as a result of diapedesis. The appearance of the retinal vessels is of great prognostic importance in evaluating hypertension and are probably more important than the manometer readings themselves. The appearance of a Grade 3 or Grade 4 fundus is of serious import but can be reversed by appropriate medical therapy. The point to be emphasized is that one should never treat a patient with hypertension without following the retinal blood vessels. Because many of the visible vessel signs can be partially or completely reversed by treatment, it is difficult to assess how much of the observed change is organic and how much is due to vessel spasm. Treatment is in the domain of the medical physician.

Arteriosclerosis

As mentioned before it may be impossible to separate hypertension from arteriosclerosis since the two often run hand in hand. Futhermore, it is possible to have one without the other. The first signs of arteriosclerosis are probably the so-called involuntary sclerosis in which the vessel walls become straight, narrow and pale. At first this may be patchy and, again, it may be rather widespread within the fundus. If it is not treated, there follows a stage during which there are caliber variations of the blood vessels, plus the arteriovenous crossing changes, which we have previously discussed. This in turn is followed by a retinopathy consisting of hemorrhages and soft spots and, finally, the malignant form of hypertension with papilledema. The papilledema is not an arteriosclerotic manifestation but is a manifestation of severe hypertension. A copper-like and silver wire appearance are arteriosclerotic manifestations.

The literature tends to divide arteriosclerotic retinopathy into a *dry form* and *wet form*. In the *dry form*, there is an essentially normal looking optic nerve but the vessels exhibit arteriosclerotic changes of various degrees. We may see numerous tiny white spots scattered throughout the retina with evidence of obliteration of retinal vessels with cystoid or cobblestone degeneration in the periphery of the retina. The latter may lead to retinal tears and retinal detachment. The *wet form* is that which is associated with tremendous edema and transudation within the retina plus the development of deep choroidal or deep retinal hemorrhages. These are eventually replaced by fibrous tissue, resulting in a fibrous tissue pseudotumor in the macular region called a Kuhnt-Junius or disciform degeneration of the macula or pseudotumor of the retina. Peculiarly enough, this is one of two retinal manifestations of Paget's disease, the other being angiod streaks. The complications of arteriosclerotic retinopathy are arterial and venous occlusions, and a vascular form of papilledema.

Patients who have arteriosclerosis often have other evidences of systemic disease. The arteriosclerosis in the fundus may not mirror initially arteriosclerosis elsewhere in the body but eventually it is a fairly reliable guide to the vascular state of the rest of the body. Patients with retinal arteriosclerosis may or may not have cerebral arteriosclerosis but often exhibit cerebral manifestations.

Spasm of the vessels, which is called an angiospastic retinopathy, is a frequent concomitant of malignant hypertension and may originate as on a renal disorder. The chief characteristic of this condition is a marked attenuation or narrowing of the retinal arterioles. It has already been stated that, while the central artery of the retina is a true artery, its branches are arterioles. Since there is marked sluggishness of the retinal circulation, the entire fundus appears pale and ischemic. Papilledema is a frequent occurrence in this condition and flamed-shaped hemorrhages and cotton wool spots are frequently present. When edema, cotton wool spots or other transudates occur in the macula, a macular star will be present.

Temporal Arteritis
Temporal arteritis is a systemic disease which commonly manifests itself with a palpable, tender temporal artery and a sudden blindness on one side which eventually may be followed by sudden blindness on the other side. There is an elevated sedimentation rate. The retinal picture is one of ischemic optic neuritis. The disc is edematous, the arteries are narrowed, but hemorrhages are usually lacking.

The treatment consists of intense, immediate treatment with large doses of corticosteroids. The proof of the diagnosis is a histologic picture of a giant cell arteritis of the biopsied vessel.

Diabetic Retinopathy
Diabetes is one of the more common of the systemic diseases. The retinopathy occurs in almost every patient after approximately 12-15 years of diabetes. It is a discouraging retinopathy, which may markedly affect vision at a time when the retinopathy ophthalmoscopically appears to be minimal. Most commonly it consists of minute, round red spots which are microaneurysms, often occurring in grapelike clusters. There are also larger, round "bullet-shaped" hemorrhages occurring within the interstices of the retina. The aneurysms are succeeded by soapy or waxy, small white, fairly hard spots or plaques, which occur around the macula and tend to form circinate figures. The spots may coalesce. Later we often see new blood vessel formation around the optic nerve, over the

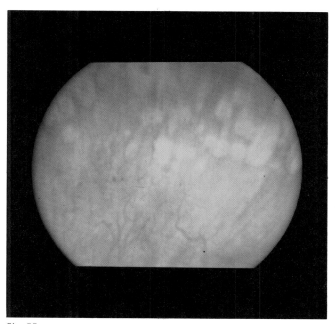

Fig. 55
Cobblestone degeneration of the retina. Found in the far periphery.

Fig. 56
The angiod streak on nasal side of the disc is a dark blood vessel-like streak which goes down along the disc. This is not a vessel but is blood vessel-like (angiod) in appearance and due to a crack in the glass membrane of the choroid. Angiod streaks occur in Groenblad-Stranberg syndrome and Paget's disease.

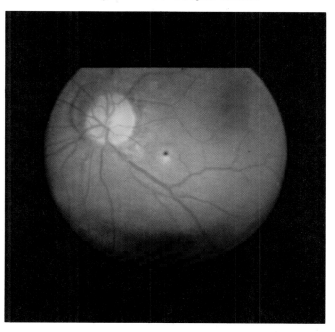

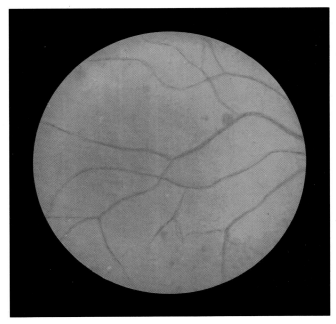

Fig. 57
Aneurysms in a diabetic. Note the tiny red dots near blood vessels. The larger blotch-shaped red area is probably a hemorrhage.

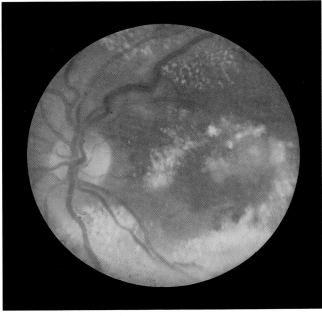

Fig. 58B
Diabetes, later stage than Fig. 58A, with massive transudates, many of which are blurred because of the heaping up with local edema—patient has Kimmelsteil-Wilson's disease.

Fig. 58A
Classical diabetic retinopathy. Waxy golden transudates with a circinate configuration. The aneurysms tend to occur in grape-like clusters.

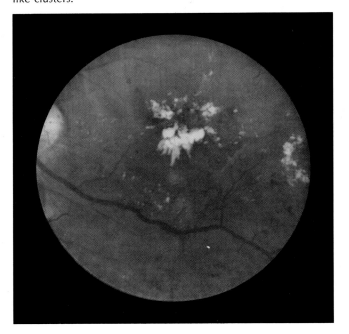

Fig. 59A
A late stage of diabetic retinopathy showing a large vitreous hemorrhage in front of the retina. There are newly formed vessels in thin sheaths or veils on the retinal surface and in the vitreous.

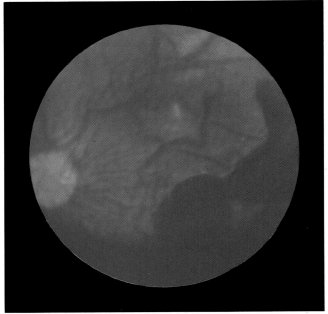

retina and into the vitreous, together with fine veils over the retina and frequently vitreous hemorrhages. The vitreous hemorrhages absorb rapidly at first, and more slowly or not at all later. In the process of absorption, fibroblastic and angioblastic tissue is formed, creating strands of fibrous tissue over the retina and into the vitreous. At this stage retinitis proliferans is present.

Aneurysms are usually found near retinal veins, and are often difficult to visualize unless a fluorescein stain is used. Aneurysms by themselves do not cause any effect on vision. Later they may result in retinal edema and as previously stated in the production of the soft, waxy exudates. These exudates do affect vision and may cause either a marked decrease in vision or tiny scotomata. While they are most significant when occurring in the macular area, they do tend to occur on the nasal side of the disc and the mid-periphery of the retina. Initially, exudates are seen on either side of the disc, especially on the temporal side. Cotton-wool spots are also seen in diabetes, although not as commonly as the waxy exudates. Originally it was hypothesized that cotton-wool spots indicated hypertension but this is not necessarily the case. Hypertension may be superimposed upon a diabetic retinopathy as in the so-called Kimmelsteil-Wilson disease (Fig. 58B). In this condition a mixture of the two pictures is seen with a predominance of soft, cotton-wool spots, coppery arteries and arteriovenous compressions.

An important change may occur later in the retinal veins, with generalized dilation and localized changes in the caliber of the veins called "beading." "Beading" is seen as a fusiform dilation of parts of the veins. The veins begin to form loops and may become reduplicated with formation of shunt vessels and neovascularization on the anterior surface of the retina. The blood column begins to slow down as seen occasionally by the segmentation of the columns.

The appearance of the neovascularization on the surface of the retina, with its concomitant sheathing or veils, means that the diabetic retinopathy is now in the proliferative stage. New vessels become adherent to the retina and later begin to exert traction so it becomes detached with the traction causing the vitreous hemorrhages. All of this sets up a vicious cycle of retinal ischemia, hemorrhages, traction, detachment, and eventual blindness.

It is a tragic fact that once a diabetic retinopathy occurs its course is completely disassociated from patient control of the diabetes.

Treatment: The best treatment, of course, would be the prevention of diabetes, an impossibility at the present time. The two best treatments today are: (1) hypophysectomy, and (2) photocoagulation of the

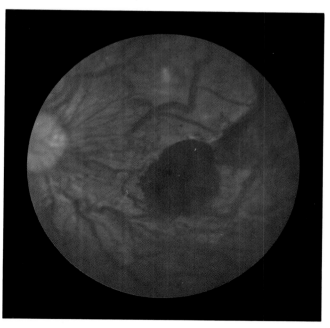

Fig. 59B
Same patient with the camera focused on the vitreous.

Fig. 60
Retinitis proliferans. This follows repeated vitreous hemorrhage. The fibrotic bands are part of the healing process.

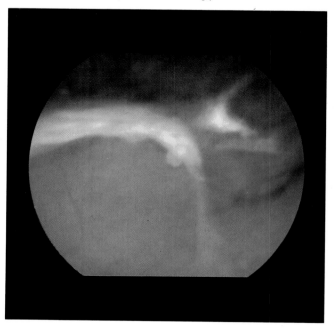

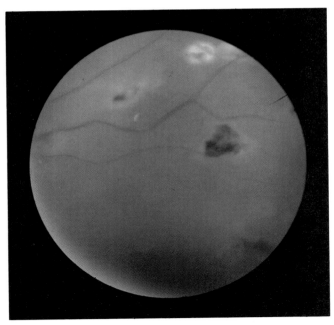

Fig. 61
Thermal choroiditis after photocoagulation of bleeding areas in diabetic retinopathy. The pigmented-depigmented areas are the sites of photocoagulation.

Fig. 62
Roth's spot—patient with septicemia. Note the large striate hemorrhage with the white center.

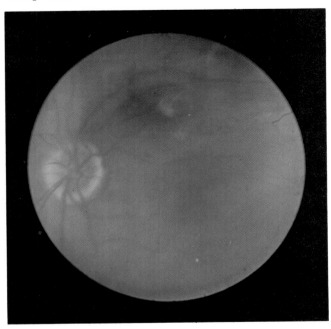

bleeding sites. The latter can be repeated as necessary as long as the photocoagulation does not take place too close to the macula. Some laser beams can be used for the same purpose. The efficiency of hormonal and anticholesterol therapy in the mitigation of diabetic retinopathy has not yet been proven.

Subacute Focal Retinitis (Roth's Septic Retinitis)
Subacute focal retinitis is found in patients already seriously ill with a septicemia, i.e., subacute bacterial endocarditis. The characteristic fundus picture is one of hemorrhages with small, round or oval white spots often situated in the center of the hemorrhages. The hemorrhages do not tend to have the boat-shaped configuration often found in leukemia and are said to be, but are not, pathognomonic of leukemia. The hemorrhages are often surrounded by edema. They occur more commonly near the disc and rarely near or in the macula. The affect upon vision depends upon the site of the retina obstructed. If a hemorrhage or transudate occurs in the macula, especially overlying the fovea, the visual effect is great. If the lesion occurs away from the macula without associated macular edema, there may be little or no effect upon vision. Roth's spots are not associated with retinal abscesses, but if a metastatic purulent embolus reaches the retina, a retinal abscess will result.

Vasculitis
Retinal perivasculitis is a rather common inflammatory occurrence and especially affects the veins (periphlebitis) and less commonly the arteries (periarteritis). The inflammation of the blood vessels is associated with hemorrhages into the retina and vitreous. These hemorrhages tend to be recurrent as long as the inflammation is present. Complications following repeated bleeding, retinitis proliferans and secondary glaucoma are seen. It must be emphasized that vasculitis is not a specific condition and has many different etiologies.

Vasculitis may be due to a uveitis, to metastases or to involvement in some systemic disorder, or may be local within the retina as in Eale's disease (periphlebitis). When uveitis causes a vasculitis, there will be sheathing and caliber changes within the artery and generally marked dilation of the veins and even papilledema. In my experience, the greatest dilation of the veins and arteries occurs in young people with posterior uveitis not associated with obvious choroiditis.

Vasculitis associated with a systemic disease would be part of that disease. The retinal picture would not be pathognomonic of the systemic disease.

Eale's disease has long been known in ophthalmology and is especially prevalent in young males, 20 to 25 years of age. The disease tends to be bilateral and the etiology is unknown.

The clinical picture involves either the peripheral veins or the central larger veins. Usually the first knowledge that the patient has of the disease is a sudden loss of vision due to a retinal and vitreous hemorrhage. During the active stage, one finds small, white exudates clustered around the affected vessels. When the lesions heal, the vessels may become sheathed. Some patients have only one or more attacks while others have repeated attacks leading to eventual blindness. When healing takes place connective tissue strands are laid down which tend to drag onto and detach the retina, similar to the manner described in diabetes.

Treatment: There is no known effective treatment, however, one can attempt to photocoagulate the bleeding points.

Coloboma of the Optic Nerve and Choroid
Partial or complete absence of the optic nerve is a congenital defect which is seen ophthalmoscopically as a cavity within the disc area and completely within the sheath of the nerve. At times, part of the nerve may be present and the rest replaced by the cavity, which is called a pit. These pits or holes appear bluish in color. The colobomas are reported to be due to a defect in closure of fetal fissure. Therefore, a coloboma, or absence of the choroid, typically lies below the optic nerve, although it may atypically occur in other sites. The defect in the choroid is seen as a

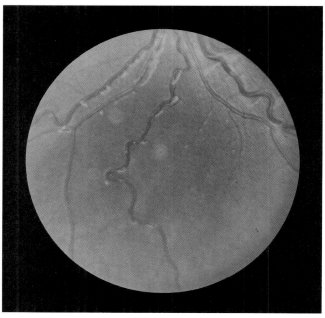

Fig. 63A
"Candle droppings" in a patient with Boeck's sarcoid uveitis. Note the discrete infiltrates against the vessel walls.

Fig. 63B
Overwhelming meningitis terminating fatally, severe perivasculitis, sheathing of the vessels with exudates.

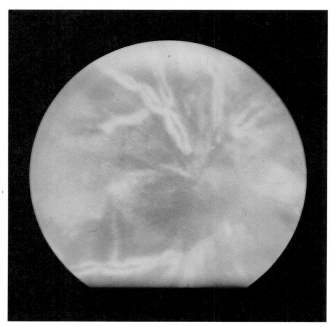

Fig. 63C
Paravenous atrophy. One set of vessels is outlined by an area of choroidal atrophy, Paget's disease.

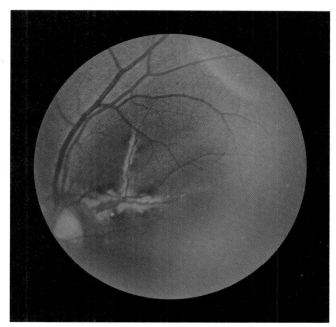

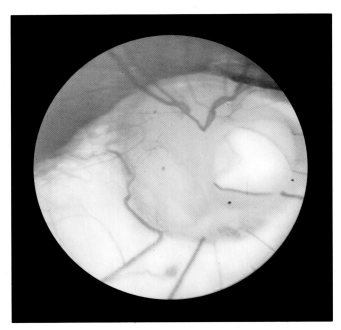

Fig. 64
Coloboma of the optic nerve and choroid occurring in the typical site of the embryonic fissure. The small red field represents normal choroid.

somewhat crescentic, white area, since one is looking at the sclera with some tissue interposed between the viewer and the sclera. Pits in the optic nerve are most commonly found on the temporal side of the disc and frequently are followed by detachment of the adjacent retina. Often the retina will later reattach spontaneously but only with a marked loss of vision. Obviously, the area of coloboma is blind. Coloboma of the choroid is frequently associated with an absence of part of the overlying lens and iris, which means that the inferior portion of the lens and iris would be absent. Coloboma of the optic nerve is associated with a marked visual defect.

Blood Dyscrasias
Blood dyscrasias include virtually all afflictions of the blood cell-forming organs including the anemias, leukemias, lymphomatous diseases, sickle cell retinopathy, polycythemia, lipemia retinalis, fat embolism in the retinal vessels as well as the blood borne exogenous toxins.

It is well known that the retina can react to insult in one or more ways, the most important being edema, hemorrhages, transudates, or areas of inflammation in which there is edema. A lesion exhibits pigmentation as part of the healing process. Hence there are few absolute pathognomonic pictures, but certain insults do tend to produce somewhat characteristic pictures.

Fig. 65A
Sickle cell disease with hemorrhagic perivascular infiltration and sheathing.

Fig. 65B
This is a terminal stage of sickle cell retinopathy, with retinitis proliferans occurring over the site of previous neovascularization.

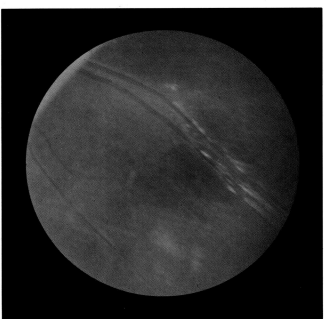

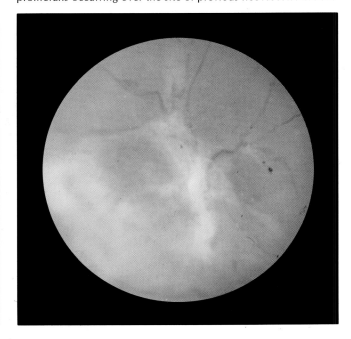

The most common characteristic seen with severe anemia is marked pallor of the optic nerve and retina and hemorrhages within the retina. The retinal hemorrhages are small and flame-shaped. The "retinal" color of red comes from the choroid which is also anemic, hence the pallor.

Sickle Cell Retinopathy

Sickle cell retinopathy occurs in sickle cell (SC) anemia. The characteristic findings are fullness and tortuosity of the retinal veins, with ischemic areas, neovascularization, telangiectasis and microaneurysms in the far periphery. Later, choroidal and retinal degeneration with capillary thrombosis and retinal hemorrhages occur. Cholesterol crystals may be present near the retinal vessels at this stage. The end point is characterized by a tremendous retinitis proliferans with hemorrhages into the vitreous with arterial and venous occlusions.

Leukemia

The retinopathy found in leukemia is not pathognomonic of either the lymphatic or myelogenous type.

The textbook picture of leukemia is one of widespread pallor with boat-shaped hemorrhages having white centers plus a marked perivasculitis. In my experience there is a marked difference in appearance between the childhood and adult types of leukemia. In childhood leukemias, one finds primarily an exudative type of disease. Therefore, exudates may appear in any part of the fundus, typically in front of the optic nerve simulating a papilledema, which also can occur. There may be exudates similar to cotton-wool spots scattered throughout the fundus. Occasionally, a child will exhibit a severe hemorrhagic retinopathy. In the adult, the large canoe or boat-shaped hemorrhages with the white centers can be more characteristic. Generally, these seem to occur most often in the shape of hemorrhages hanging from the optic nerve.

There are so many new types of treatment for the leukemias, especially in children, that the clinical picture which is described as a leukemic retinopathy may in part be due to the therapy itself.

Polycythemia

Polycythemia is characterized by a tremendous increase in the numbers of red corpuscles in the blood. As a result the exposed parts of the body, such as the face, are reddish purple in color, and the fundus tends to exhibit a similar characteristic. There will be tremendous dilation of the veins which are almost purplish in color. The fundus picture depends upon an over-production of red blood cells and, therefore, is absent when the condition is controlled.

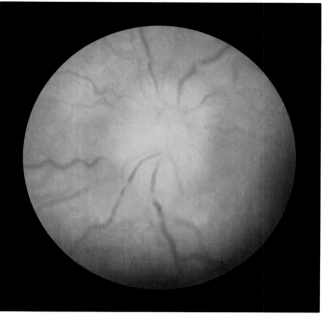

Fig. 66A
A transudate overlying a retinal vessel. This is not diagnostic, but does localize the transudate in the nerve fiber layer or on the retina itself.

Fig. 66B
Hemorrhages in the periphery of a boy with lymphatic leukemia. The hemorrhages are not pathognomonic.

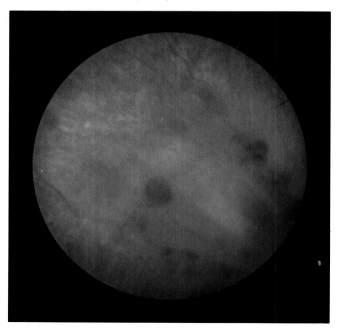

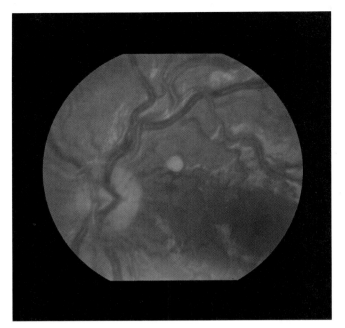

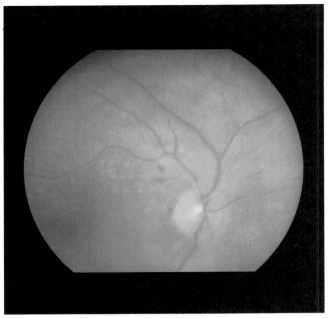

Fig. 67
Polycythemia. Tremendous engorgement of all vessels, with cyanosis of the retina.

Fig. 69A
Lipemia retinalis in a light-skinned individual. The vessels are full of fatty blood (cholesterol 1880) so that it becomes difficult to differentiate veins from arteries. The entire fundus is milky.

Fig. 68
Tetralogy of Fallot in patient with congenital heart disease. Note the engorged vessels and the purplish retinal cyanosis which matched the cyanosis of his skin.

Fig. 69B
Lipemia retinalis in a deep brunette on an abnormally high fat diet (blood cholesterol 1600). The fat-filled vessels stand out like white lines on the brunette background.

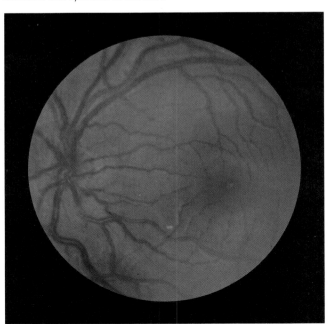

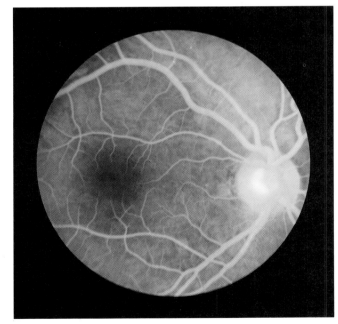

A similar picture occurs in congenital heart disease when there is a marked decrease in oxygen supply with production of the condition known as Tetralogy of Fallot. This presents itself as an exaggerated cyanosis of the entire fundus.

Lipemia Retinalis

Lipemia retinalis is due to an excess of cholesterol in the circulating blood and is found in individuals on a high cholesterol diet (often induced) or in diabetic coma. The blood vessels become milky in color, so that it becomes difficult to distinguish arteries from veins. The picture is most pronounced when it occurs in dark-complected individuals, when the almost white blood vessels stand out in sharp relief on the dark background. In lighter individuals the entire fundus may appear a milky blue in color. While most of the reported cases have been noted during diabetic coma, the majority I have seen, have occurred in patients who did not have diabetes but who were on an unusually high fat diet.

Fat Embolism in Retinal Vessels

Fat emboli may follow a fracture of one of the long bones with a fat particle getting through to the retina. Here one sees glistening particles of fat in the retinal vessels, occluding them and causing ischemic infarcts beyond the occluded portion of the artery. There is a marked similarity between this condition and Purtscher's disease which is a retinopathy due to a distant injury, commonly a crush injury of the thorax. One sees a definite edema of the retina, with hemorrhages, fat emboli and cotton-wool spots, so that it may be virtually impossible to differentiate any true fundus detail. This may clear spontaneously but usually retinal and optic atrophy ensue. A head injury may cause the identical response.

Lymphomatous Disease

There is no characteristic textbook picture of lymphomatous disease within the retina. The lymphomatous exudates may be found in the retina and look like small exudates due to other causes. They are not diagnostic. Retinal hemorrhages and exudates also may occur.

Macroglobulinemia

This is one of the dysproteinemias due to a disturbance in the reticulo-endothelial system with the presence of abnormal globulins in the circulating plasma. The clinical picture demonstrates marked venous congestion with marked dilation and tortuosity of the veins followed by hemorrhages, so profuse as to completely obscure all retinal detail. The final stage is one of actual venous occlusion. The entire picture may be reversed by appropriate treatment of the macroglobulinemia.

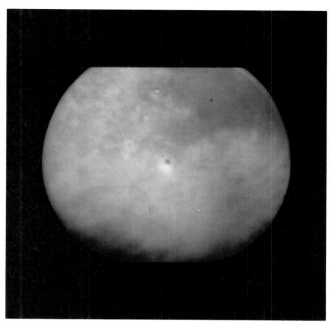

Fig. 70A
Purtscher's traumatic retinopathy following a crush injury of the thorax. The fundus is so full of edema, fat embolisms and hemorrhage, that it looks like a gray-red blur.

Fig. 70B
The same patient several months later. The retina is still somewhat edematous with a red "hole" in the macula. The eye is blind.

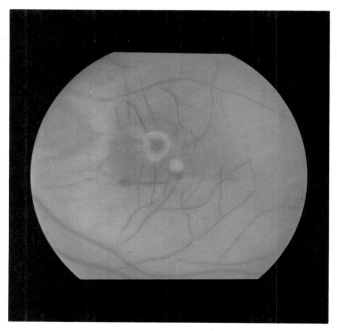

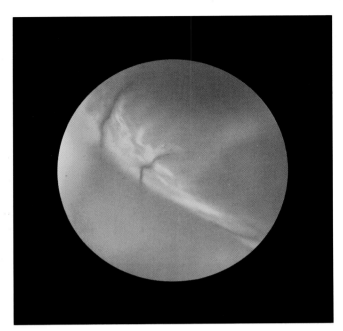

Fig. 71A
Retinal detachment viewed in front of red fundus, with a fold of retina which appears enwrapped by vessels.

Fig. 71B
A filmy band of retinal tissue (including vessels) seen in the vitreous. There is a slightly curved red streak in the elevated tissue representing a tear in the detached retina.

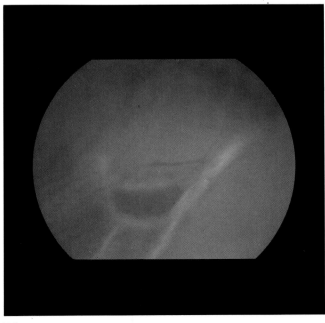

Retinal Detachment

Retinal detachment is not truly a retinal detachment, which implies that the retina separates from the choroid, but rather the pigment layer of the retina remains attached to the choroid and the rest of the retina detaches from it. This condition is almost a classically textbook or "telephone diagnosis" picture like appendicitis, in that the sequence of events almost always tends to be somewhat similar. The patient first sees "stars" and later has the sensation of a curtain moving across his field of vision. The loss of vision will depend upon the site of detachment and whether it involves the macula. If the detachment is below, the upper field of vision is lost and the patient will not be as aware of it as when the detachment is above and the lower field is lost. At times a detachment occurs simultaneously with a massive vitreous hemorrhage, which completely obscures the view of the fundus. When the hemorrhage absorbs or settles down, a retinal detachment is found. Therefore, any vitreous hemorrhage must be regarded as probably masking a retinal detachment until proven otherwise.

Because the detached retina is farther forward and closer to the observer than is the rest of the retina, it will be impossible for the examiner to visualize the detachment and retina in one ophthalmoscopic plane. Usually the picture is one of a gray or silvery billow containing black looking retinal blood vessels, floating or standing out in front of the red fundus. The detached area may seem to be stationary or may wave back and forth. It may even be thrown into folds. The detachment can be so flat as to be hardly visible excepting to the trained eye. Often the detachment will only be found with a plus-12 or 16 lens because the retina is so far forward. Careful examination reveals a small, somewhat triangular or crescentic-shaped, brilliant red area which is a so-called retinal break or tear. The red is the red of the choroid seen through the hiatus in the retina. Frequently, areas of healed choroiditis will be found in such an eye as well as other degenerative changes which are apparent only to the skilled observer. Detachments of the macula do occur but fortunately less commonly than peripheral detachments. When there is a tear or break in the macula itself, return of central vision is virtually impossible.

Malignant Melanoma of the Choroid

When the detachment has a solid appearance, one must think either of a deep, massive hemorrhage or tumor. An elevation of the retina due to hemorrhage will tend to subside when the hemorrhage begins to absorb. The detachment of tumor tends to increase and eventually the retina comes off beyond the area of the tumor so that one will see the solid appearing area in addition to a waving area in which there is shifting fluid. The trained observer will be able to note shifting fluid within a true retinal detachment. Metastatic lesions, as from a breast cancer, usually cause flatter, yellow detachments.

Nevus of the Choroid (benign melanoma)

Malignant melanoma of the choroid must be differentiated from benign melanoma or nevus of the choroid. The latter is usually seen as a small, dark, slatey blue lesion appearing slightly elevated and which lies under the retinal vessels. At times, there are tiny, white, calcium flecks on its surface but at other times it will appear to be dusky brown in color. The color is usually more vivid than a malignant melanoma which is usually dull grey in appearance.

The benign melanoma does not cast a scotoma in the visual field and apparently never becomes malignant. It is more sharply defined in its borders than is a malignant melanoma. There are some flat densely-pigmented malignant melanomas which in the beginning look like huge nevi. However, the malignant melanoma, when observed, will grow, and detach the retina above and around it.

Retinoblastoma

Retinoblastoma, a comparatively rare tumor, is the most common intraocular tumor of young children. It is first noticed because of the yellow or cat's-eye reflex seen in the youngster's pupil. Ophthalmoscopi-

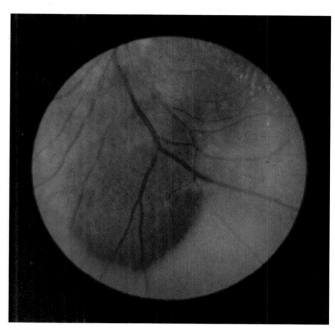

Fig. 72A
Malignant melanoma of the choroid. One sees a huge, blue-black area which does not appear to be elevated.

Fig. 72B
A solid looking gray retinal detachment with vessels climbing over its surface. This is a malignant melanoma of the choroid until proven otherwise.

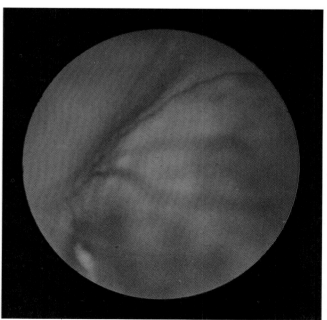

Fig. 73
A yellow, slightly elevated area above the optic nerve in a patient with advanced carcinomatosis due to a breast lesion.

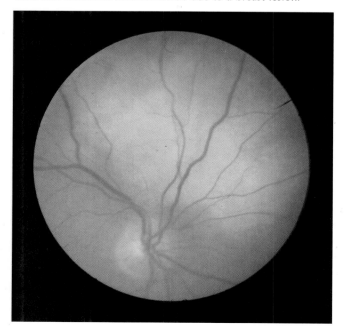

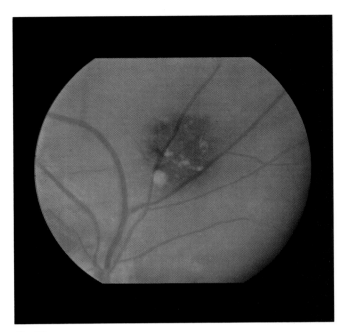

Fig. 74
Benign nevus of the choroid. This does not elevate the retinal vessels.

cally one sees the early lesion as an elevated, white area, usually in the midperiphery. There are frequently multiple tumors as they tend to seed other areas. Neovascularization or calcification may appear on their surfaces. Much of the retina may be detached as the lesions progress. Strabismus may be the first clue to the lesion, as with other visually disturbing intraocular diseases of infants and children.

Pigment Anomalies
There are many pigment anomalies of the retina and choroid. Any insult in the way of disease, trauma or inflammation of either of these structures must affect the pigment layer with resultant proliferation, atrophy, disappearance or heaping up of the pigment. Pigment may clump or pile up over the optic nerve, usually on the edges, giving the appearance of a pigmented tumor. The pigment may form unusual configurations within the retina or the choroid. Little is known about the choroidal pigment. There is a condition called melanosis oculi in which the pigment may appear in sheets in any part of the eye. In another condition known as congenital grouped pigmentation of the retina, the pigment is found in small, round, noninflammatory dots scattered primarily in one quadrant of the eye. It has been described as looking like "bear tracks," rarely affects both eyes and does not affect vision. Whenever an inflammatory lesion oc-

Fig. 75A
The cat's-eye reflex from the pupil of an infant with retinoblastoma, which can often be seen when the light strikes the pupil.

Fig. 75B
Retinoblastoma—a common intraocular tumor of infancy, seen as a large white mass elevating the retina.

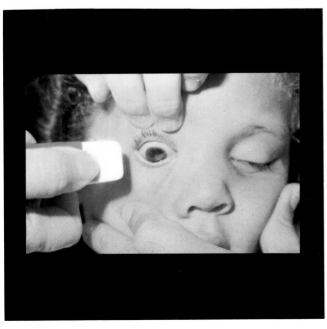

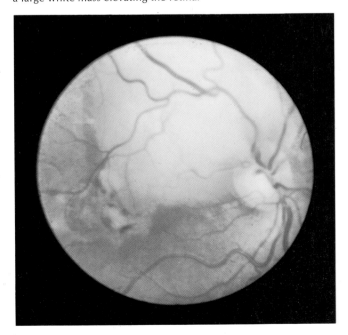

curs in the choroid or retina, part of the healing process involves pigment moving into the lesion and surrounding it. Clinically the appearance of pigment within an inflammatory lesion heralds the healing of the lesion.

Retinal Schisis
Retinoschisis occurs most typically in hyperopic young males with a splitting of the two layers of the retina. The inner layer of the retina which carries the large blood vessels, becomes translucent and usually is perforated with one or more large spaces. There is a frequently associated atrophy of the choroid but this rarely results in retinal detachments. However, the possibility remains and these patients must be carefully followed. The condition is thought to be hereditary. It is commonly seen in the lower temporal quadrant of the eye and is frequently symmetrical in both eyes. A scotoma results. When it occurs in the lower part of the retina, the scotoma would be projected superiorly where it is often not noticed.

The Macula
Inasmuch as the macula is the center of the finest detailed vision, afflictions of this area are of extreme importance. The macula is subject to the same diseases and tumors as may occur anywhere else in the body. In addition there are a number of dystrophies

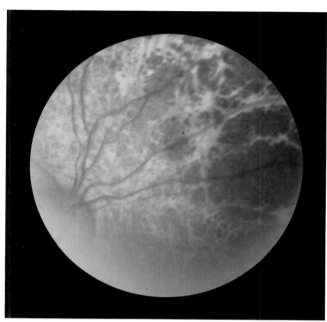

Fig. 76A
Melanosis oculi—a densely pigmented fundus with no affect on vision.

Fig. 77
Retinoschisis in one quadrant with the retinal blood vessels climbing over the abnormal area. The latter is split and has four torn areas through which the underlying remaining thinner retina is visible.

Fig. 76B
Congenital grouped pigmentation. This is without significance.

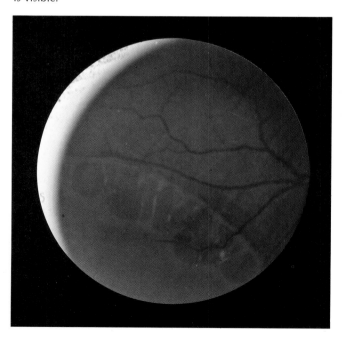

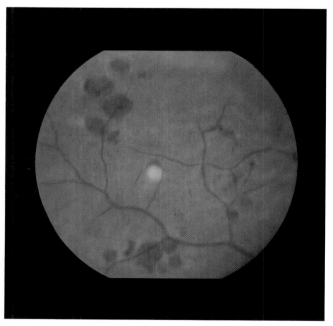

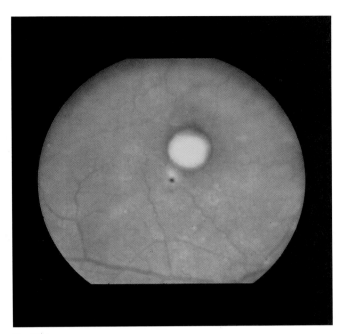

Fig. 78A
Vitelline degeneration of the macula termed "fried egg, sunny-side up."

involving the macula, especially in the older age group, that have a definite deteriorating effect upon vision. Any lesion which destroys macular elements markedly affects vision. The same type of lesion occurring in the periphery or mid-periphery of the eye, would have little or no observable effect upon vision. While there are no blood vessels directly in the center of the macula and the fovea, there is a rich blood supply around the macula. Macular transudates tend to assume a circular configuration.

Because the retinal nerve fiber layer of Henle radiates away from the fovea, the typical macular star will occur if there is edema or transudation within the macular area. Surprisingly enough, a star-shaped configuration of a macular hemorrhage is almost never seen.

Central Serous Retinopathy (Angiospastic Retinopathy)

An edema of one macula is a fairly common occurrence in young or middle-aged individuals, usually males, under extreme nervous tension. It is also often found in individuals who are heavy cigarette smokers. The characteristic feature is edema of the macula, which appears to be elevated and around which there is a circular reflex which does not shift with the motion of the ophthalmoscope, i.e., it does not disappear. The retinal vessels around the macula will appear to be spastic, however, this is not always the

Fig. 78B
Sjogren's reticular dystrophy.

Fig. 79
Circinate retinopathy thought to follow a deep retinal or choroidal hemorrhage or associated with intraocular helminth.

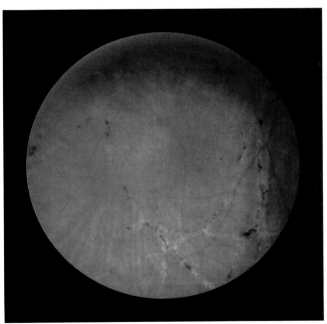

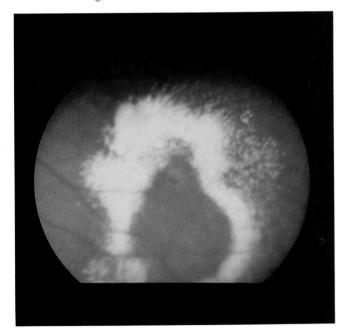

case. When these lesions subside they may leave pigment dots or white deposits behind. The effect upon vision may be minor or great. When fluorescein studies of the eyes are done, small choroidal leaks are usually found. After photocoagulation the patient receives a permanent cure. Most patients clear up spontaneously but may have future recurrences which also spontaneously disappear. Photocoagulation is done only in cases of long standing which do not exhibit evidence of improvement. Simply stopping smoking may result in a cure or it may occur after corticosteroid therapy. Angiospastic retinopathy should not be confused with a malignant melanoma of the choroid.

Macular Holes and Cysts

A small, cystic degeneration of the macula, primarily occurring in the fovea, may follow trauma, inflammation, or may come on without any apparent reason. The usual picture is a small, sharp, red circle in the center of the macula which has a pigmented appearance and may resemble a nematode egg when seen under the microscope. These lesions are referred to as "holes" or macular cysts. They have a markedly destructive effect on central vision. Sometimes the top layer of the retina, i.e., the layer nearest the ophthalmoscope, will come off and be seen floating around in the vitreous as a small bluish-grey operculum. This rarely produces a retinal detachment.

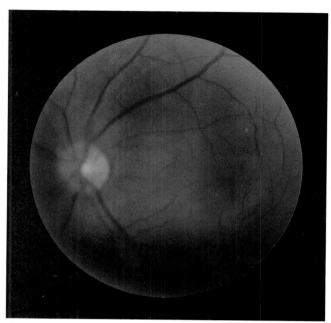

Fig. 81A
Cyst or hole formation in the macula. Note the bull's-eye of a mottled, reddish circle surrounded by a halo.

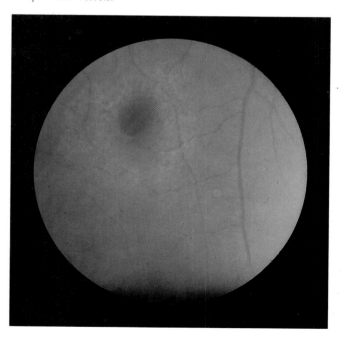

Fig. 80
Central serous retinopathy, (dark central area) surrounded by a lighter circular area of retinal edema (almost cherry-red) with fairly normal vessels.

Fig. 81B
Macular cyst. Observe the round lesion just under the terminal edges of the inferior macular vessels.

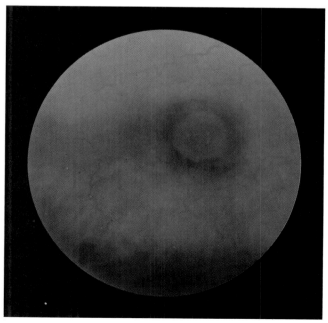

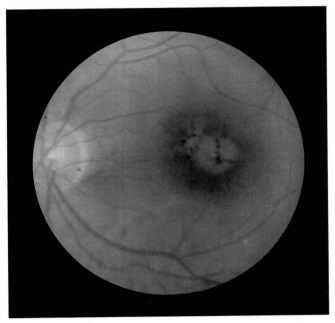

Fig. 82A
Senile macular degeneration—pigmentation and depigmentation of the macula in the aged.

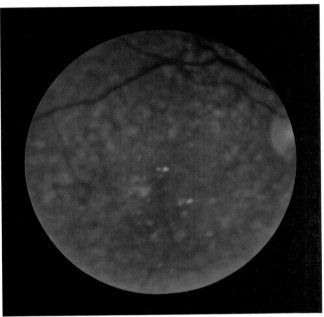

Fig. 82C
Drusen (colloid degeneration) of the retina. The myriads of round, white dots are deep to the retinal vessels. The glistening golden dots are cholesterol.

Fig. 82B
Early senile macular degeneration showing loss of normal macular detail.

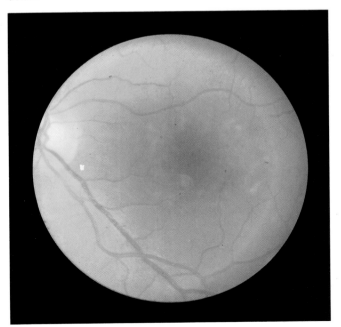

Fig. 83
Central areolar choroidal sclerosis. Note the sharply demarcated central circle, absence of macular detail and the white choroidal vessels.

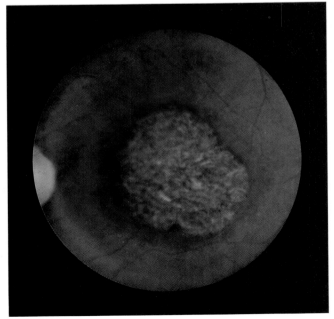

Senile Macular Degeneration

Degeneration of the macula may occur at any age but is more common in the elderly with tragic results upon the central vision. The characteristic appearance is a blotchy and deep pigmentation of the macular area. This is difficult to visualize during the early stages and when photographed, reveals almost no evidence of disease because the ophthalmoscopic change is so slight at this time. As the degeneration progresses the pigment clumping and stipling with the simultaneous depigmentation and pallor in this same area becomes more marked. There is an obvious loss of color vision with the formation of a central scotoma. The visual loss may be far in excess of the lesion, and conversely a sorry looking macula may have surprisingly good vision. Rarely there may be sclerosis of the choroidal vessels in the macula as well as elsewhere. In this situation we see what appear to be white, anastamotic blood vessels which take on the configuration of the superimposed layers of the choroid. The choroidal vessels do not anastamose but since there are several layers heaped up over each other, the appearance on the flat section (with the ophthalmoscope) is that of an anastamosis or interlacing network of vessels; when white in color, it is called "choroidal sclerosis."

An appearance similar to that of senile macula degeneration is seen in a group of conditions which are hereditary and which may occur at any age, including the young. These conditions take on various appearances, but fundamentally, pigmentation and depigmentation are characteristic. This book will not attempt to confuse the observer by detailing the various forms of senile, juvenile, or hereditary macular degeneration. Edema and hemorrhage may be concomitant features of macular degeneration although the occurrence of hemorrhage is much less than pigmentation, depigmentation, or edema. At times heredomacular degeneration may be associated with cerebral degeneration.

Tumors in the macula do not differ from tumors elsewhere within the retina. This same statement applies to inflammations and injuries within the macula.

Choroiditis (Choroidal Inflammation)

Inflammations of the choroid are a part of the broad picture of uveitis. The choroidal inflammation may occur in any part of the globe and manifests itself initially by a marked loss of vision especially if it occurs in or near the macula or it may not affect vision appreciably if it appears at a distance from the macula. If the inflammation is large it will discard sufficient inflammatory products into the vitreous so that the patient will see many spots and will be bothered by them. When seen ophthalmoscopically, the early,

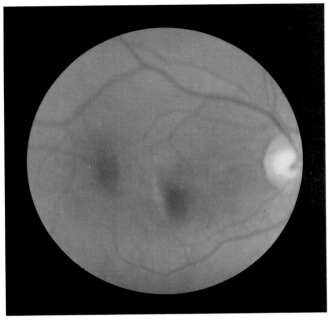

Fig. 84A
Male, who was "mugged" shows choroidal rupture in the macula and marked loss of central vision. A crescentic rupture is parallel to the optic disc.

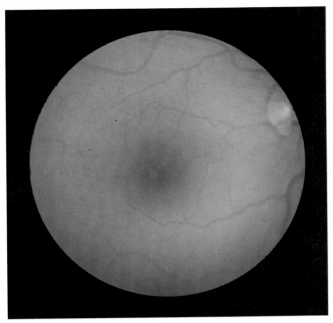

Fig. 84C
Mild eclipse burn of the macula. The foveal reflex is replaced by a round pale (burned) area, surrounded by a darker circular zone.

Fig. 84B
Huge choroidal rupture following severe trauma to the globe. Such a rupture is always concentric to the disc.

Fig. 84D
Neuritis papulosa—a triad of neuritis, choroiditis and periphlebitis often due to syphilis.

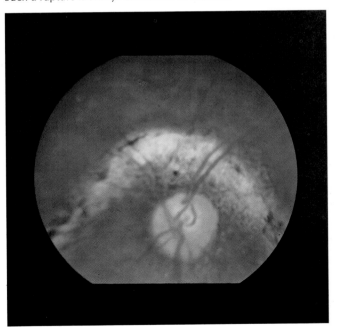

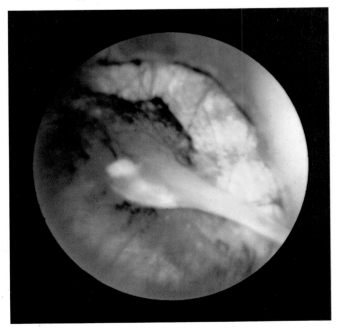

active choroiditis appears to be a raised, yellowish area within the fundus. If the area of choroiditis is large, the amount of exudates poured forth into the vitreous will render ophthalmoscopy almost impossible. However, the observer will usually see a yellowish area which will be the cue to the diagnosis. When one looks into a fundus whose media is so hazy that detail is impossible to visualize, it will usually be possible to see the orange, yellowish appearance of the optic nerve. This is seen best when the patient is looking directly ahead. However, if two yellowish lesions are seen, one can be differentiated as the optic nerve, and the other as an area of choroiditis. Or, if the yellow area is not in the position of the optic nerve, it obviously must be a lesion of some sort. When the choroiditis is treated by corticosteroid therapy, it begins to flatten down, fundus detail becomes more visible, and the vitreous haze begins to disappear. As the lesion heals and flattens out, it becomes white as the destruction of the choroid renders the underlying sclera visible. At the same time, pigmentation occurs around the borders and within the healing lesion. The end result is that of a white pigmented lesion. There are several characteristic features. Toxoplasmosis causes a characteristic picture, in which there is initially one large area of choroiditis, often in the macula. Recurrences tend to occur adjacent to the initial lesion and actually hook onto it forming an appearance which we term "satellite lesions." The end result may be a large lesion, obviously composed of several smaller ones. Similar large lesions may occur elsewhere within the globe.

Secondly is that which we term "presumed histoplasmosis." Here we find small, scattered lesions with typically a lesion in the macula and other lesions adjacent to the optic nerve (juxta papillary). The macular lesions tend to be surrounded by tiny caps of hemorrhage. The small hemorrhages tend to be recurrent and destroy the macula, resulting in fibrous tissue proliferation with a somewhat heaped up scar.

In the third picture, which will not be evident to the unskilled observer, there are lesions far out in the periphery of the retina near the ora serrata. This is a so-called "pars planitis" because it occurs in the region of the pars plana. However, these distant lesions tend to produce macular edema and marked loss of central vision. There are also associated fibrous tissue masses, usually in the lower pole of the fundus and most prevalent in females. These masses look like white detachments or elevations or even pseudotumors. Since they are far down in the periphery, they may be difficult to visualize. However, unexplained macular edema and loss of central vision simultaneously appearing with many vitreous opacities should lead one to suspect pars planitis.

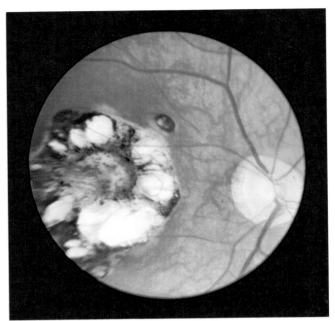

Fig. 85
Choroidal scars in the macula. This is the classical picture of toxoplasmic choroiditis with many conglomerate scars due to one lesion hooking on to the site of a previous one.

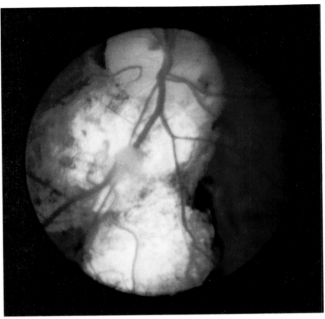

Fig. 86B
Toxoplasmic chorioretinitis similar to Fig. 86A, with conglomerate scars of more than one lesion hooked together.

Fig. 86A
Toxoplasmic chorioretinitis with an active lesion (soft, fluffy, poorly focused) to the left between the disc and macula.

Fig. 86C
Acute toxoplasmic retinopathy. This is a periphlebitis with a yellow-white pigmented veil between the bifurcating branches of a vein.

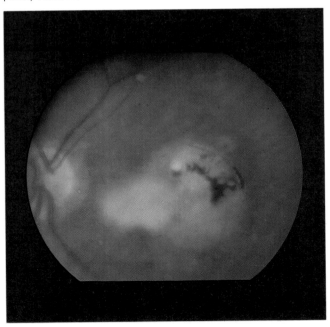

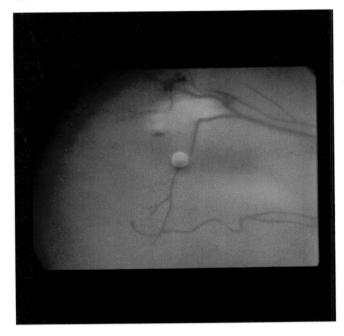

Tapetoretinal Degenerations (Abiotrophies)

There is a large group of retinal-choroidal conditions which are known as *tapetoretinal degenerations* because they affect that part of the retina and choroid which is the site of the tapetum in canines and other animals. These conditions are practically always hereditary, even though the mode of inheritance is unclear. Fundamentally, they produce changes in night vision and later in day vision with scotomata in the visual field. Few of these patients go completely blind, but as they become older many suffer marked loss of vision and restriction of the visual field. The most characteristic field defect in this group is the so-called ring scotoma. When one carefully plots out the visual field in patients with early retinitis pigmentosa and early choroideremia, characteristically a series of rings or anular scotomata either partially or completely circumscribing the field will be found. These tend to increase in number and in width as the disease progresses and coalesce, so that the anular configuration disappears as the field itself becomes lost.

Essentially these dystrophies fall into two broad groups: (1) in which pigmentation is a marked feature and (2) in which pigmentation is not a marked feature. Often the two forms seem to be co-mingled

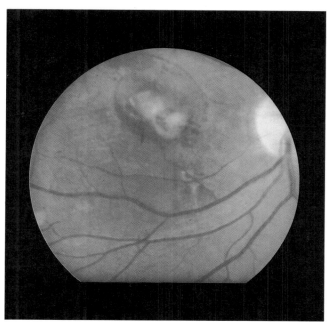

Fig. 87B
"Presumed histoplasmosis"—a later stage than Fig. 87A, with a healed (hard, easily focused) lesion, surrounded by a cap of hemorrhage.

Fig. 87A
"Presumed histoplasmosis" with a small yellow lesion in the macula, beginning to pigment (healing) and a macular star-like area of edema around it.

Fig. 88
Ring scotomata in a patient with retinitis pigmentosa. The black areas are the blind zones in the field.

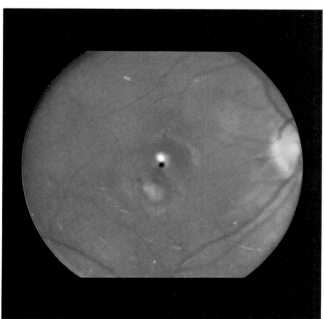

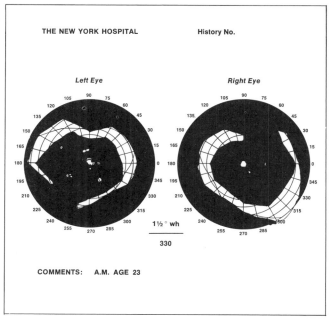

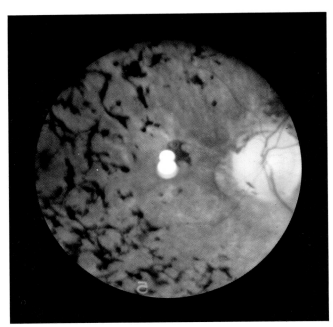

Fig. 89A
Retinitis pigmentosa. Spidery pigment corpuscles in the perivascular spaces with white atrophic disc and narrowed blood vessels.

Fig. 89B
Drusen of the optic disc composed of concentric laminations of hyaline material. They sometimes appear faceted or numular.

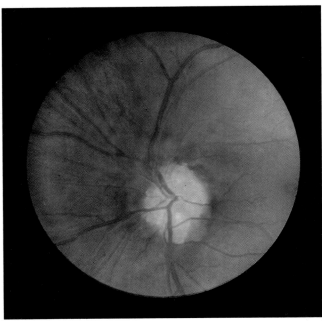

within the same patient. At times more than one type of retinal abiotrophy will be found within a single family.

The best known member of that group in which pigmentation is a prominent feature is retinitis pigmentosa. Retinitis pigmentosa is practically always an inherited disease and may be acquired via a dominant, recessive, or sex-linked mode of transmission. The patient first notices difficulty in moving about at night, and later, as the field defects progress, begins to bump into people and objects during the daytime. This is followed by a marked loss of visual field and eventually loss of central vision. At the same time, many of these patients begin to develop posterior subcapsular cataracts.

When one views the fundi of these patients, vitreous opacities are present and, at times, large vitreous cysts. About 2 to 3 percent will exhibit a persistent hyaloid artery. The disc becomes dirty-white in appearance; the retinal arteries become sclerotic and narrow. Many of these patients exhibit a dark, slate grey tesselation. Eventually, spidery pigment corpuscles appear first at the nasal mid-periphery and later scattered throughout the fundus in association with the retinal veins. The pigment may also be seen cuffing some retinal arteries. Pale atrophic patches appear within the fundus. The choroidal circulation may become visible and even sclerotic. Faceted diamond-shaped lesions may appear on the optic nerve. These lesions are referred to as drusen of the optic nerve. At times they may seem to spill down from the optic nerve into the retina. There may be tiny white dots interspersed with the pigment dots.

Choroideremia

Choroideremia is a condition affecting only males and transmitted by the female carrier. Essentially symptoms are similar to those of retinitis pigmentosa and when early choroidal atrophy begins and is accompanied by dispersion of choroidal pigment, the picture may be confused with retinitis pigmentosa. The female carriers of the disease exhibit pigment clumping usually in the mid-periphery but have no significant visual disturbance. There is a slow progressive atrophy of the choroid without involving the macula until almost the end of the disease. As the picture eventuates, the optic nerve and the macula stand out as two reddish elements within a sea of white.

Retinitis punctata albescens

There is another night-blinding disease whose symptoms resemble retinitis pigmentosa but which is characterized by innumerable tiny white dots scattered throughout the fundus. It occurs in two forms: (1) in which all of the symptoms resemble those in retinitis pigmentosa and, (2) in which the symptoms are observable by the patient only in dim light. He has no trouble in good light. As stated before, this condition and retinitis pigmentosa may seem to coexist in the same patient.

Gyrate atrophy of the Choroid

This is a rare condition of the same night-blinding family and is characterized by escalloped areas of choroidal atrophy with a large white necklace of sclera occurring either around the optic nerve or out in the mid-periphery. These areas of choroidal atrophy coalesce and increase with eventual loss of vision and even blindness. When the areas of white sclera become massive, the remaining choroid stands out sharply as red islands in the sea of white.

Phakomatoses

This is a group of five diseases, probably inherited, in which there is an association of somewhat similar lesions in the skin, central nervous system and eye. Most of the patients exhibit more than one sign of the disease, although it is rare to find all of the signs in any one individual.

The members of this group are: (1) Tuberous Sclerosis (Bourneville's disease), (2) Neurofibromatosis (Von Recklinghausen's disease), (3) Encephalotrigeminal angiomatosis (Sturge-Weber disease), (4) Retinocerebellar angiomatosis (Lindau-von Hippel dis-

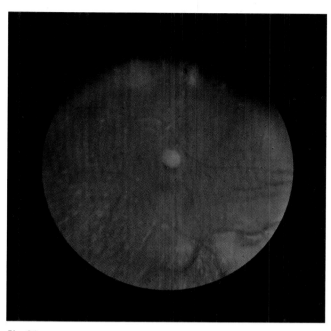

Fig. 91
Retinitis punctata albescens. Note the white dots (elongated appearance) lying deep to the retinal vessels.

Fig. 90
Choroideremia—progressive atrophy of the choroid with night blindness. The disc and retinal vessels appear to be normal. The choroid is slowly atrophying and the sclera (white) is becoming visible.

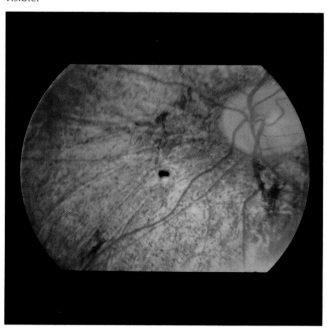

Fig. 92
Gyrate atrophy of the choroid. Note the escalloped areas of choroidal atrophy with some shreds of red choroidal tissue in the atrophic areas.

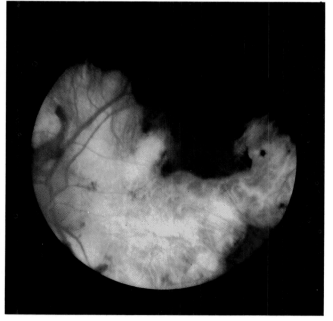

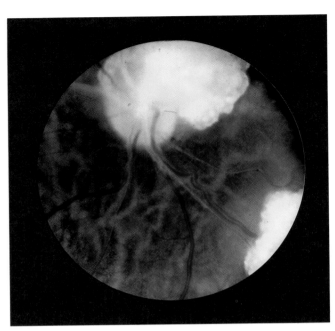

Fig. 93
Tuberous sclerosis with two gliomas (astrocytic) of the nerve and retina. A large white faceted (mulberry-like) mass is coming off the upper disc. A similar lesion can be seen down in one corner of the field.

ease), and (5) Familial telangiectasis (Osler-Rendu disease).

Bourneville's Disease (Tuberous Sclerosis)

This condition has a classic triad of symptoms; adenoma sebaceum, most commonly confined to the face but also seen elsewhere, epilepsy and mental deficiency. Most of the cases reported have not exhibited mental deficiency. It is usually manifested early in life among females. One may also see congenital tumors of the retina, kidneys and heart, which are referred to as tubers. Spina bifida, polydactyly, microcephaly, and high arched palates have been reported, as well as rhabdomyoma of the heart, also have been reported. As a rule, many of these patients die in their late teens or early twenties. The skin lesions seen are multiple, smooth, red or pink nodules in the butterfly area of the face, chin, and occasionally on the forehead and scalp.

The most characteristic lesion within the eye consists of small tumors or tubers which are faceted and which may be pedunculated. They are often found in association with the optic nerve but may occur elsewhere in the eye. When one finds such a lesion, studies should include encephalograms, X-rays of the skull and long bones and electrocardiograms. These ocular lesions grow slowly and consist of a proliferation of astrocytic cells which arise in the nerve fiber layer of the retina.

Neurofibromatosis (von Recklinghausen's disease)

This syndrome exhibits skin manifestations varying from the well known cafe-au-lait spots occurring on the small of the back, but more common on the thighs, plus hard, rubbery subcutaneous nodules which may occur anywhere on the body and are termed neurofibromata. Neurologic manifestations are a common part of this disease because of the occurrence of the neurofibromata in the central nervous system. The latter lesions are usually gliomas of the brain and the optic nerve. Neurofibromata in the lid are a common cause of ptosis in children.

Occasionally one may see tiny, raised "freckles" on the iris. These are local manifestations of the disease. Lesions similar to those seen in von Recklinghausen's disease may also occur within the retina. Another common finding is persistent medulation of the retinal nerve fibers. These may be small astrocytic tumors rather than the medulation which they mimic. The most important ocular finding of neurofibratomatosis is a glioma of the optic nerve or chiasm. Usually these lesions become apparent early in teenage. There is a common triad of unilateral loss of vision, proptosis and optic atrophy. When the tumor occurs within the optic nerve out of the ophthalmoscopic range, it will produce papilledema. Characteristically, the optic foramen is enlarged on X-ray.

Encephalotrigeminal Angiomatosis
(Sturge-Weber disease)

This condition characteristically includes an unilateral nevus flammeus on the face, although it may be bilateral and associated with large cavernous hemangiomas. It is reported that when it involves the distribution of the first division of the trigeminal nerve, glaucoma always occurs on that side. This has not been uniformly true in my experience. The important fact is that glaucoma is frequently found on one side and that the appearance of this lesion on an individual's face demands careful examination and observation for glaucoma.

Often, when these patients are first seen, the disc is already glaucomatous. There may be an associated hemangioma of the choroid, which is seen as a dark area within the choroid, moderately elevated and often speckled with white dots. If the hemangioma is tiny, it may be missed. Similar lesions within the brain produce central nervous system symptoms.

Retino-cerebellar Angiomatosis
(Lindau-von Hippel disease)

This disease is characterized by cysts and tumors of the abdominal wall, kidneys, pancreas, plus angiomatosis of the cerebellum and retina. Calcification in the brain and the retina is commonly seen on X-ray. Involvement of the central nervous system may result in increased intracranial pressure, headache, nausea, vomiting and papilledema as well as staggering, dizziness and nystagmus. Often, if the lesion occurs in the cerebellum, it will not occur in the retina and vice versa.

Angiomas of the retina are usually present at birth but may go unnoticed because of their tiny size. These tend to grow and are usually detected in late teenage. In about half of the patients angiomatosis of the regina is eventually bilateral. At times the lesion will first be found in one eye and a thorough search will fail to reveal any other lesion. Later in life other lesions will be noted. The textbook picture is that of an artery and vein coming together in the mid or far periphery to produce a small to large aneurysm. Frequently tiny benign-looking, orange lesions are found scattered in the mid or far periphery. There may be one or several when the patient is first examined. Later, other similar lesions develop. The lesions may bleed, producing the appearance of a white, dirty painted retina. Considerable bleeding will produce vitreous hemorrhage and obscuration of fundus detail. Growth of the lesions without treatment (photocoagulation or freezing) results in retinal detachment unresponsive to therapy. The angiomatosis may involve the optic nerve with a vascular lesion at this site. Frequently, in angiomatosis as well as in others

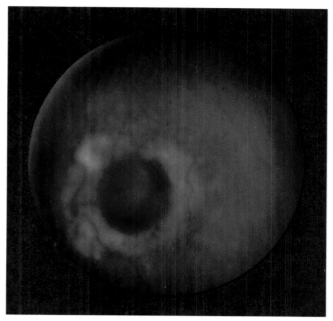

Fig. 94A
An arteriovenous aneurysm in a patient with Lindau-von Hippel disease. The artery and vein come into the circular aneurysm in the far periphery of the retina.

Fig. 94B
An aneurysm in the far periphery of a boy with Lindau-von Hippel disease.

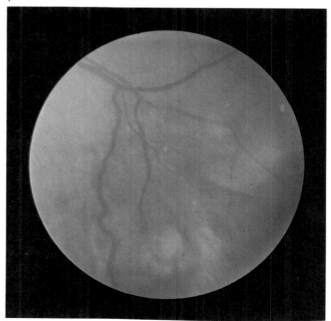

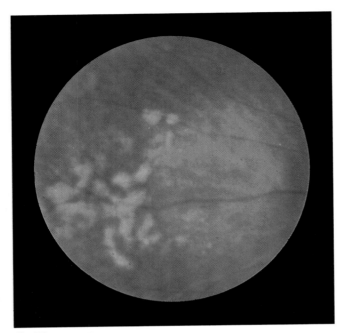

Fig. 95
Osler-Rendu disease (familial telangiectasia). These soft white lesions are confined to one quadrant of one eye and resemble "Drusen."

of the group of phakomatoses, a family history of similar lesions will often be obtained.

Familial Telangiectasia (Osler-Rendu disease)
This is characterized by telangiectases which are usually spidery in appearance, occurring on the face, within the nose, on the conjunctival surface of the lids, and other mucous membranes. Characteristically, many of these patients have recurring nose bleeds, whose etiology may at first escape the physician. This disease is more common than realized, probably because the symptoms are usually minimal. However, bleeding may occur from any mucous membrane including the gastrointestinal tract and can result in death. The characteristic intraocular lesion is either a telangiectasis of the retina which may resemble that on the mucous membranes, or a discreet aneurysm. These aneurysms may become closed off and appear like a collection of retinal drusen. This should not be confused with ataxiatelangiectasia (Louis-Bar syndrome). The latter occurs in young children in which spidery telangiectases are seen on the face and eyes, with associated strabismus, ataxia and death at an early age.

Conclusion
Guidelines to ophthalmoscopy have been laid down. The interpretation of ophthalmoscopic findings should be facilitated by applying these observations under clinical conditions. A number of nerve and chorioretinal diseases have been briefly described in an attempt to orient the student in the world of the ocular fundus. It is a very interesting world to the ophthalmoscopist who has made an effort to learn his way around it.

Suggested Bibliography

1. Ballantyne, A. J. and Michaelson, I. C.: *The Fundus of The Eye.* Williams and Wilkens, Baltimore, 1967.
2. Davis, M.: The Natural Course of Diabetic Retinopathy. *Trans. A.A.O.O.* 72:237, Mar.-Apr. 1968.
3. Duke-Elder, S.: *System of Ophthalmology.* Vol. II, The Anatomy of The Visual System. Henry Kimpton, London, 1961.
4. Duke-Elder, S.: *System of Ophthalmology.* Vol. X, Diseases of The Retina. Henry Kimpton, London, 1967.
5. Durham, R. H.: *Encyclopedia of Medica Syndromes.* Hoeber-Harper, N.Y.C., 1960.
6. Gass, J. D. M.: Phakomatoses. in Smith, J. L.: *Neuro-Ophthalmology,* Vol. II, C. V. Mosby, St. Louis, 1965.
7. Lieber, B. and Olbrich, G.: *Klinischen Syndrome.* Urban and Schwarzenberg, München, 1966.